RENEWALS 458-4574
DATE DUE

FEB 17			
ILL:	629580S	AHH	
	JUN 2 6 2003		
	NO RENEWALS		

GAYLORD PRINTED IN U.S.A.

STRATEGIES FOR INTEGRATED HEALTH CARE

STRATEGIES FOR INTEGRATED HEALTH CARE

Emerging Practices in Information Management and Cross-Continuum Care

Erica Drazen
Jane Metzger

Foreword by Scott Parker

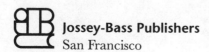

Jossey-Bass Publishers
San Francisco

Jossey-Bass books and products are available through most bookstores. To contact Jossey-Bass
directly, call (888) 378-2537, fax to (800) 605-2665, or visit our website at www.josseybass.com.

Substantial discounts on bulk quantities of Jossey-Bass books are available to corporations,
professional associations, and other organizations. For details and discount information, contact
the special sales department at Jossey-Bass.

Manufactured in the United States of America on Lyons Falls Turin Book. This paper is acid-free
and 100 percent totally chlorine-free.

Library of Congress Cataloging-in-Publication Data

Drazen, Erica.
  Strategies for integrated health care : emerging practices in information management and
cross-continuum care / Erica Drazen, Jane Metzger ; foreword by Scott Parker. — 1st ed.
    p. cm.
  Includes bibliographical references (p.   ) and index.
  ISBN 0-7879-4159-X (acid-free paper)
  1. Integrated delivery of health care. 2. Information resources management.
I. Metzger, Jane. II. Title.
  RA971.6 .D72   1999
  362.1'068—ddc21

98-40134

FIRST EDITION
HB Printing   10 9 8 7 6 5 4 3 2 1

CONTENTS

FOREWORD

The pace of change in health care is not abating. Those of us who work in this field face a seemingly endless parade of challenges as we work toward a truly seamless care relationship with our patients that consistently produces good outcomes. We have come to know firsthand that we must move quickly. We no longer have the luxury of addressing change in a reactive mode or implementing change on an incremental basis. We must move decisively and boldly—or we may find ourselves too far behind the curve to recover.

We can take some comfort in knowing that we are not alone in this dilemma, but that does not help with the task at hand. Learning critical lessons about process and organization from one another, however, can be the lever that each of us needs to address the challenges of true integration. This book is a classic example. I am proud of the participation of Intermountain Health Care in the two major research collaborations reported in this book. Understanding the similarities and differences among health care organizations, and sharing successes in process improvement, can help us collectively reduce risk and enable more rapid transformation to truly integrated care management.

The authors of this book performed an invaluable service when they asked a small number of health care organizations to join with them in taking a look at emerging practices in integrated health care. They brought the vision and perspective of well-informed researchers, but came only with the intent to listen and learn, and to increase everyone's understanding. The results of their queries are in the pages that follow this foreword. The authors provide a very practical look at the new processes that the organizations they studied are creating and what it takes—in organization and information management—to be successful. Their pragmatism shines through in the introduction as well, which thoughtfully guides those of us who are pressed for time. I commend the authors for their clear-eyed look at emerging practices, I commend the organizations that openly shared in and facilitated this work, and I trust that this book will inspire you in your efforts to improve care and service for those you serve.

May 21, 1998   Scott Parker
Salt Lake City, Utah   Chief Executive Officer
                                                          Intermountain Health Care

ACKNOWLEDGMENTS

This book reflects contributions from dozens of people who participated in the research and worked behind the scenes to make the preparation and publication of this book possible. To list everyone would take pages, but some deserve special thanks.

Our primary sponsors in this endeavor were Jim Reep, the CEO of First Consulting Group, and Stan Nelson, Chairman of the Scottsdale Institute. They were certain of our success long before we were and gave us unwavering support through all stages of the project. We could not have done this without their visionary leadership in both this project and their respective organizations.

This book reports on the results of two collaborations. We would like to acknowledge the time and enthusiastic support of the primary collaborating organizations. First we would like to thank those who worked with us on the integrated delivery network (IDN) of the 21st Century:

Larry Grandia, Sherry Monson, and Belle Rowan of Intermountain Health Care

Robert Pickton and Pat Johnston of Baylor Health Care System

John McDaniel and JulieAnn Wright of McLaren Health Care Corporation

David Pryor and Joanne Sunquist of Allina Health System

Terry Carroll and Marge Matthews of Detroit Medical Center

Staff from many other sites shared their experiences and contributed knowledge that allowed us to define new models and create an overall framework for understanding them. Without their help the project would have been less efficient and less successful. Special thanks also go to Teresa Fama, deputy director of the Chronic Care Initiatives in HMOs, for a thoughtful review of our work on new models for cross-continuum care management.

A second group of leading IDNs contributed staff time and lessons learned to the information technology (IT) benchmarking collaborative, reported in Chapter Nine. They were willing to try "one more time" to get useful benchmark metrics. They have also helped share our findings by participating with us in presentations at industry meetings. We are grateful to the following:

Judy Botwick (former CIO), University Medical Center, Tucson

George Conklin (former CIO), Integris Health

John Glaser, Partners HealthCare System

Larry Grandia, Intermountain Health Care

Mike Minear, HealthSystem Minnesota

Dave Selman, ProMedica Health System

Rick Skinner, Providence Health System

Tommy Bozeman, North Mississippi Health Services

Bertram Reese, Sentara Health System

Norm Smith (former CIO), Henry Ford Health System

We quickly learned that collaborative research differs from the research approaches we had used before. Maureen Bisognano and Penny Carver of the Institute for Healthcare Improvement and Gordon Mosser and John Sakowski of the Institute for Clinical Systems Integration functioned as a virtual collaborative research "support group." We thank them all for sharing common challenges and helping us discover more effective approaches to our work.

Protocols or guidelines integrated into clinical decision making are key elements of the new models for the IDN of the 21st Century. Three vendor organizations graciously shared their protocols and guidelines, giving us permission to incorporate them in the scenarios in Chapters Five and Eight and in a demonstration tool we have developed to illustrate how new process models and IT converge for IDN providers and patients on a day-to-day basis. We owe special thanks to the following:

Nancy Whipple, Rosemary Sheehan, Paul Brient, and Andrew Garling of HBO & Co. (formerly HPR, Inc.) for use of a care strategy from the Clinical Care Management System®, and for assistance with a case scenario demonstrating how the care strategy's assessment, stratification tool, and time-sensitive interventions guide the case management process

Numerous individuals at Access Health for use of a telephone triage algorithm from FirstHelp®

Gordon Mosser of the Institute for Clinical Systems Integration for the use of a care guideline for simple cystitis developed and implemented by ICSI member organizations in Minnesota

Many of our colleagues at First Consulting Group participated in the on-site data collection, in synthesizing the results, and in reviewing drafts of this book. Other colleagues have used the results of our initial projects in the field and shared their experience. Their feedback has improved the packaging of our findings and added greatly to our knowledge in these emerging areas.

A special thanks is due to Kevin Smith of First Consulting Group's help desk, who rescued chapter drafts from our hard drive on at least two occasions when we thought they had vanished forever! Two Barbara's—Barbara Kendall and Barbara Wyse—were brave enough to help us through the preparation of a second book (though they knew better). They played an equally important role this time around, keeping us and our piles of reference materials organized, improving clarity and packaging, riding herd on version control, and always moving ahead, even when the task appeared overwhelming.

Andrew Pasternack, our editor at Jossey-Bass, displayed the appropriate balance of urgency and forgiveness to keep the book on schedule, while enabling us to continue in our "real" job of applied research.

Despite this long list of contributors, the driving force behind this book was Jane Metzger. She urged us to consider formally publishing our research findings, actually wrote two-thirds of the chapters herself, and kept us going when we all thought better of the idea. Her family (husband George and daughters Erica and Lisa) also deserve recognition. They certainly remember that after the last book we did pledge "never again!" Nevertheless, they endured interrupted family plans and living amidst piles of book materials one more time.

Of course we must end by thanking our clients and colleagues in the industry who have always been willing to give us opportunities to learn and share, and settings in which to experiment. They make our work both possible and very rewarding.

May 1998   Erica Drazen
Boston, Massachusetts

ABOUT THE AUTHORS

ERICA DRAZEN is vice president of Emerging Practices at First Consulting Group (FCG), where she runs the applied research function. Previously, for twenty-five years she was a consultant and researcher at Arthur D. Little. The focus of her research has been innovative applications of information systems in health care, with a special emphasis on evaluation of benefits. She was the principle investigator on NCHSR projects to evaluate patient monitoring systems, computerized electrocardiogram analysis systems, and hospital information systems, and on DoD-sponsored evaluations of pilot clinical systems and the Composite Health Care System. Through the years she has provided leadership to the CHIM, the College of Healthcare Information Management Executives, and the Computer-Based Patient Record Institute (CPRI).

JANE METZGER is vice president of Emerging Practices, the applied research arm of FCG. Previously, for twenty-five years she did consulting and research on patient care processes and on the integration of information technology (IT) at Arthur D. Little. A special area of interest is patient care processes, especially ambulatory care, and how to rethink and empower them with IT. At FCG she has worked on understanding new enterprisewide processes of integrated health systems, including access to care, cross-continuum care management, and deploying best practices. Metzger is a founding member of the CPRI work group that organizes and runs the Davies Recognition Program for Excellence in CPR Implementation.

INTRODUCTION

Erica Drazen

This book is intended to meet the needs of those who lead efforts to integrate care and thus provide new levels of performance in our health care system. This certainly includes those who are trying to build clinically integrated systems of care. Clinical integration requires redesigning and sometimes even totally rethinking the way care is accessed and delivered. The number of people who must participate in this change is enormous. This book is intended to provide an introduction, a framework, and some practical advice for the participants.

The core of the book describes the new models that organizations are designing and implementing for accessing and managing care across the continuum—processes that are on the agenda of almost every health care institution in the country. Obviously, accessing and managing care are two of the core processes in care delivery; they involve patients, providers, and administrators and they touch almost every part of a care delivery organization. The book takes the perspective of the delivery system, although the concepts presented are drawn from both payer and provider organizations. The lessons learned are applicable to all organizations that strive to improve access to care and to better manage the care of patients.

We hope that all participants will gain insights from this book that will help them move more quickly and with fewer missteps along the way. The executive level of management will gain an understanding of the magnitude of the change ahead and familiarity with critical success factors and benefits so that they can become knowledge leaders and promoters of the transition to new models of care delivery. Managers who make the change happen will receive some practical advice and guidance. Information systems managers will gain a jump start on evolving process models and their information challenges. Suppliers (especially of information systems) will gain insight into the requirements they will be asked to support.

We realize that we are addressing a broad audience. We have also come to appreciate the complexity involved in creating truly integrated care delivery systems. This book does not skimp on details. However, we have tried to apportion the discussion into chapters that will be of broad interest and chapters that will be of greatest interest to those "in the trenches."

This book is about information management, which includes the design of both the processes and the information systems that make these new processes work. The focus on information technology reflects our heritage as authors and the recognition that clinical integration requires advanced information systems support. To make the technical requirements clear to all readers, we have made generous use of scenarios and illustrations of the type of information systems that participants in these new processes would actually use.

How We Came to Write the Book

The content of the book came primarily from the results of research conducted by the Emerging Practices Institute, which is the applied research function of First Consulting Group. As with most research efforts, the path had a few unexpected bumps and turns; however, the essence is quite straightforward. We recognized the fact that the pace of change in the health care industry will continue to accelerate. Our clients were also accelerating their investments in health care information systems. This combination of factors increased the risk involved in planning for information systems (one of our core businesses). One of the greatest risks was that investments made today would not be effective in meeting tomorrow's needs.

The goal for the research program was simple: identify emerging approaches to information management and emerging technologies that had the potential to create significant value for the health care industry. Once these emerging practices were identified, our mission was to build the knowledge and skills needed to help our clients plan now so that they will be able to use these emerging approaches effectively in the future. We also wanted the knowledge to enable our clients to be as aggressive as they desire in implementing advanced approaches.

We defined a few principles for the research program:

- Research would be conducted in collaboration with health care industry leaders who were ready to experiment and to pilot new approaches and who were willing to share their experience with us and with the industry.
- We were committed to applied research—in the broadest sense of the concept. We would select research areas with high relevance to future needs and do our research at actual practice sites. We also wanted to package our research findings so that they could easily be applied in the future.
- We would address the broad topic of information management—the underlying business strategies, the necessary process improvements, and the required organization and governance, as well as the enabling information technology.
- This would be a continuous process—we would develop frameworks to make it easier to add to the knowledge base and share information in the future.
- Finally, we decided that we would share the knowledge we gained with clients and the industry at large. This book is one part of that effort.

Why We Picked These Research Topics

While doing our market research we became aware of the confusion in the market about definitions. What was this integrated delivery network (IDN) we were seeking? How would we know when a delivery network had become truly integrated? And perhaps most important, how did we know whether the actions we were taking today were leading us in the right direction or creating barriers for the future? After a quick review of existing research (see Chapter One), we set about creating a definition of the IDN and the processes that would create integration.

We were lucky to cross paths with another group, the Scottsdale Institute (SI), then called the Center for Clinical Integration. The SI members are senior executives (chief executive officers, chief information officers, and chief medical officers) of integrating delivery systems. The founder of SI is Stan Nelson, who spent eighteen years building the Henry Ford Health System. He understands what is needed to create effective integrated delivery systems, recognizes that information systems are critical to integration, and is a strong believer that collaboration is a way to make faster progress toward the goal of integration.

Members of the SI helped us refine our definitions and use them to create a profile of the current status of integration. (The results are reported in Chapter One.) A subset of the SI membership also agreed to collaborate with us in defining a process framework for the future. This project was dubbed the "IDN of the 21st Century." The preliminary framework is described in Chapter Two. Many of the processes we defined did not exist in 1996, but elements had begun to emerge. We knew that we needed to gain experience with these processes to build knowledge about key success factors and benefits and to refine the details of the process framework.

Working with members of the SI, we selected two processes for our initial research focus: access to care and cross-continuum care management. These processes were selected because of their importance and because they were being planned or implemented in our collaborators' organizations. (We knew that adding a project to the organization's agenda was not feasible—our research had to fit their priorities.) As our research progressed, we discovered that these processes are often chosen as the first care processes for major "rethinking" in the integration process.

Access to care is a critical measure of system performance from a patient's perspective. A system is not viewed by patients as integrated unless they can get in to see a provider when they feel that is necessary. Cross-continuum care management represents the core business process for an IDN, and all organizations struggle to eliminate barriers to seamless care delivery across multiple settings.

We took a multistep approach to researching these emerging integrated models for care. First, we identified sites that had already experimented with some elements of a new model in the selected areas (for example, within access to care they may have implemented cross-continuum scheduling or a nurse triage service). Information was collected on these sites' experiences and from the experience of our collaborating partners to develop a framework for thinking about new models for care. This experience helped identify which elements of new models were constant, which varied, and the reasons that different sites took different approaches. It was then communicated to teams within our collaborators' sites, who incorporated the experience into their evolving designs and then provided us with additional insights.

Most of the early focus of the collaborating teams was on redesign of process; however, we also identified information and information systems requirements to support the rollout of these processes beyond a pilot stage. We also developed what we refer to as visualizations—essentially, demonstration software that helps illustrate how computers could support the different participants in the new models of access and care management. These visualizations are helpful in supplementing paper descriptions because they bring the new processes to life. We have used screen shots from these demonstration systems to illustrate changes in the roles of care providers as well as changes in information requirements.

Although most of this book deals with process change, we conclude with a chapter on information management. None of the new models for access to care or cross-continuum care management can go very far beyond planning without new information systems. The changes involve more robust infrastructure, new applications, coverage of a broader geography, and meeting the needs of new users. All of this puts a hot spotlight on the process of managing information systems and the performance of information systems departments.

The topic of best practices in information management actually came onto our research agenda at about the same time as our work on access to care and care management. Organizations were concerned about whether or not their information systems function was prepared for the challenges ahead, whether they were more or less efficient than comparable organizations, and how high-performing organizations achieve their success. Everyone recognized that the old rules used to assess the performance of the information management function in hospitals no longer applied. The industry was starved for metrics to use in comparing the performance of IDNs. There were even more questions about how to achieve high performance— What were the key baseline requirements and the secrets to success?

We developed a framework for collecting information on performance metrics and best practices and set out to find answers. We identified ten IDNs that had established track records in both building an IDN and successfully implementing the technology to support integration. These became our "learning laboratory." After days of on-site data collection and months of follow-up to fill in gaps and resolve questions, we rewarded the participants with a retreat where we discussed and extended our findings. The results of this initial effort (and subsequent additions to the framework) are discussed in Chapter Nine.

As our research proceeded, we learned about how collaborative research differs from more traditional research approaches, and we also shared "best collaborative research practices" with other collaborative research groups. That could be the subject of an entire book—our bottom line is that collaboration in all things, including research, is the future. There is too much to do in a limited time frame with too much risk involved to ever gain knowledge fast enough if it is done one person at a time. We hope our research results help you to gain some momentum in achieving your goals for creating a delivery system for the twenty-first century, and we hope you let us know about your successes and your lessons learned.

How to Navigate the Chapters

Chapter One is intended to provide the marketplace context for the later material. It attempts to sort through the discussion of virtual integration, vertical integration, and other buzzwords to define the core attributes of an integrated delivery system. It is essential reading for those who are not living through this change on a daily basis, it may be helpful for some who are, and it will cheer up those who think they are far behind the industry.

Chapter Two describes the process framework for thinking about new models of care. We suggest that all readers skim this chapter, because the remainder of the book is oriented toward future care delivery processes.

Chapters Three to Five and Six to Eight are a matched set describing the new models for access to care and cross-continuum care management, respectively. Chapters Three and Six answer the questions, Why are organizations making these changes? What is really changing? and Why do models vary? They are required reading for all and may be enough for readers who just want an introduction to the subject.

Chapters Four and Seven describe in detail the information requirements of the new access and care processes. These chapters will be of help to chief information officers and their staffs and are must-reads for all industry suppliers. Once organizations decide to move toward implementing these new approaches, those involved in the change process can benefit from understanding the information needs (and barriers).

Chapters Five and Eight present scenarios of the new processes and feature illustrative screen shots of the information support that participants in the process would require. The combination is intended to bring the process to life for executives, as well as for those who are deeply involved in process design and implementation. Of course, understanding how IT enables the process is essential for information systems professionals.

Chapter Nine contains insight into the new style of information management that will be required to support all the wonderful processes and systems discussed in the prior six chapters. Our experience indicates that the lessons learned can help executives inside and outside of the information technology field understand what the business and information systems department staff must do to create the high-performing IS function required for an effective twenty-first century health care delivery system.

CHAPTER ONE

INTEGRATING THE HEALTH CARE SYSTEM

Erica Drazen and Stan Nelson

Our health care system no longer consists solely of hospitals, clinics, independent physician practices, home care agencies, long-term care facilities, and other distinct care providers. Today we have integrated delivery networks, or IDNs.

One example is in Boston, where the signs at the former Deaconess and Beth Israel hospitals now say CareGroup East Campus and CareGroup West Campus. Baptist, Mount Auburn, Waltham, Nashoba, and Glover are also CareGroup hospitals; there are many CareGroup community (physician) practices, and the network continues to grow.

In Oklahoma, Baptist Hospital became Baptist Health System and then Integris Health. Today the system encompasses fifteen hospitals, rehabilitation centers, physician clinics, mental health facilities, and home health agencies throughout the state. Collectively, the entities in the Integris system maintain more than 1,700 licensed beds and have more than 1,200 physicians on staff. About 60 percent of all Oklahoma residents live within thirty miles of an Integris health facility or physician.

These enterprises (and similar organizations throughout the United States) would more accurately be described as *integrating* rather than *integrated* networks. They are still forming new organizational structures, organizing and delivering care in new ways, and using different metrics to measure success. Many observers argue that the phenomenon is not new: Geisinger Health System, Henry Ford, and the Kaiser System have been "integrated" for decades. These organizations, however, are also part of the current trend; for example, Geisinger has merged with Hershey to form Penn State Geisinger Health System.

Whether recent or longstanding, integrating health care is an important trend today. This chapter sets the stage for a more detailed discussion of how advanced health care networks are reinforcing that trend by integrating their operations.

One barrier to a productive discussion is that there is no consensus on the definition of what constitutes an IDN. There is even debate about whether the term should be *delivery network* or *delivery system* and whether financing of health care is integral to an IDN, and there is growing debate about whether inpatient beds are necessary to achieve true integration. The IDNs we discuss in this book have some common characteristics: They intend to deliver coordinated clinical services across a large geographical area, and they include multiple sites for care delivery (with a minimum of inpatient and primary and specialty outpatient care). This description forms our (minimalist) working definition of an IDN.

We begin the discussion with some historical context by outlining the development of the Henry Ford Health System, one of the early pioneers of the movement. Next we discuss the driving forces behind integration of our delivery systems and try to shed some light on the current debate about the requirements for integration. Finally we introduce a tool that we developed to measure integration in terms of its key processes. This process view of integration will recur throughout the book, because it is processes, not legal structures, that deliver the integration that affects outcomes of care from the patients', the providers', and the payers' perspectives.

The Henry Ford Health System Story

The Henry Ford Health System has developed as a broad-based, integrated system. Its starting point was in 1971, after Detroit had suffered a mass exodus of its population to the suburbs. This exodus began during the 1950s and accelerated after the riots and civil disturbances of 1967. Tens of thousands of citizens moved out of Detroit, and they were followed by physicians and other health care providers, as well as entire hospital organizations.

This demographic upheaval prompted the leaders of Henry Ford Hospital (which was located in the downtown area) to examine its options and begin an aggressive plan to deploy ambulatory care to its defined market (4.5 million people spread across southeast Michigan). The initial steps included building facilities and developing programs for two major ambulatory care centers (75,000 square feet) located in the suburbs of Dearborn and West Bloomfield, Michigan. These centers, opened in 1975, provided a wide range of services that included primary and specialty physicians, as well as outpatient surgery, twenty-four-hour emergency, laboratory, radiology, pharmacy, physical therapy, and dialysis services. Early on, subspecialty clinical services were provided by rotating physicians from the main hospital and clinic to the satellite centers on an as-needed basis.

These major centers immediately began to expand the scope of their services and the extent of their clinical specialization. This was followed rapidly by the development of other ambulatory centers that varied in size and the range of clinical services offered. By 1980 more than thirty such centers existed, permitting a regionalization of centers wherein referrals from primary and secondary care centers were made to the major ambulatory care centers or, ultimately, to the main clinic and hospital in Detroit. The goal was to have 90 percent of the patients within a twelve-minute drive of a care access point. An early lesson learned was that accessibility, convenient parking, and user-friendly facilities were important; many patients who had refused to go to the main clinic and hospital in Detroit returned to the Henry Ford System after several years' absence. The primary objective of the ambulatory care system was to provide an essential component of the continuum of care in a convenient manner, not to generate admission to the main hospital. It was viewed corporately as a distinct and important functional division and received high priority in terms of capital resources and a dedicated management team.

With the continuing growth and success of the ambulatory care system, the notion of adding a financing component to the system was explored. A feasibility study by the consulting staff from Kaiser-Permanente indicated that an HMO might succeed (although the lack of population growth and the high penetration by Michigan Blue Cross Blue Shield were definite negatives). In 1979, with the support and cooperation of the United Auto Workers and the Ford Motor Company, the Health Alliance Plan (an HMO) was formed. Almost immediately a remarkable synergy between the health plan and the ambulatory care system was noted. Each grew much more rapidly because of the other. It was possible to cross-market each entity to the benefit of the total enterprise. Compounded growth rates of 18 to 20 percent were experienced for several years in a mature market with no population growth. By the end of 1988 the Health Alliance Plan membership had reached 400,000, and in 1997 it exceeded 500,000.

To round out the system, other components of the care continuum were developed: Home Care Services became an important program, and two extended-care facilities were acquired through a merger with Cottage Hospital of Grosse Point.

As they developed the system, the Henry Ford executive team learned the value of market research. The communities in which they acquired or built facilities had different populations who had different needs and used different services. In a community with a growing number of young families, one priority was to develop pediatric services and offer evening hours. In another stable community with an older population, facility location (convenient to public transportation) was important. The Henry Ford team learned early that they had one care system but many variations in that system at the local level.

Although the driving force behind the growth of the Henry Ford Health System was somewhat unique, some of the lessons learned remain familiar today:

- A truly integrated delivery system benefits from a full continuum of services that have sufficient scale, balance, and geographic coverage to meet the needs of its market.
- Large-scale integration results in services that are mutually supportive and synergistic.
- The most successful IDNs have components that are successful in their own right.
- Customer service is an important basis of competition.
- Although an IDN may cover a large area, it must still customize its offerings to meet the needs of each distinct community.

Driving Forces for Integration

Fortunately, most inner-city hospitals are thriving today, and many of our cities are undergoing a revival. We are not in the crisis of Detroit in the 1950s and 1960s. It is therefore logical to ask, What are the driving forces for integration today? Where is the value? Why should we go though all this change? A few scenarios may help answer these questions:

- You notice a new pain in your shoulder that does not seem to ever go away. Should you bother the doctor about it, and if so, which doctor? Should you try acupuncture? If you do, will it be covered by your insurer?
- You go to the physician for a routine visit and she suggests that you see a specialist. To your relief, she recommends two doctors in your health plan who are excellent. When you call, however, you find that neither of these physicians can see you for three months—their new appointments are all booked! Do you wait, or should you go to another physician, one who is not on the "excellent" list?
- You go in for preoperative tests, and the first stop is a registration desk where you give information on where you live and work, your next of kin, your insurance coverage, and so on. You wonder why the hospital did not get all that information from your physician's office and why you have to repeat this information an hour later in the laboratory, and then again in the radiology department.

- Your primary care doctor refers you to a specialist in the group for further evaluation and tells you to come back in two weeks to discuss the specialist's report. When you come in for the follow-up appointment, not only is the specialist's report not back but your entire medical chart has disappeared. You schedule another appointment in two weeks and hope they will have found everything by then.
- Your elderly mother has been bothered by depression for several months. You finally convince her to see a doctor, who thinks a new drug on the market will help. When you go to the pharmacy, however, you are asked if your mother is on any medicine that might cause interactions with this new wonder drug. You know she takes several medications, but you are not sure what they are; you have no idea whether the doctor has already checked this out. You are back to square one, trying to convince Mom to go back to the doctor again.
- You are recuperating from minor surgery when the mail arrives with a bill from a physician you do not even recall ever seeing. This is the fourth bill you have received. Is this really your bill? What is it for? Is this the final bill or will there be more?

These scenarios illustrate some of the driving forces for integration. Our current health care system is "broken"; it is well designed to treat acute episodes of disease, but it is not designed to manage a patient's health. It is not only patients who worry about the disconnects in care; providers are also concerned because they cannot provide optimal care, and the unnecessary repeat tests, visits, and paperwork consume time that they could be spending with patients. Employers, who pay much of the cost of health care, are concerned that uncoordinated care and its effect on mounting costs will interfere with their ability to compete in the global economy. The government, which also faces an ever-increasing health care bill, is concerned about affording care for those who are currently covered by public programs, as well as expanding coverage to the uninsured.

Once integration begins in a market, it often moves rapidly. Of course the managed care contracting and cost pressures tend to affect an entire market. As new market forces begin to be felt, organizations often feel the need to "circle the wagons," to band together for protection. Changes as significant as those created by a managed care environment are a major impetus for change. Another accelerator of integration is the fear of being left out, especially in markets with an oversupply of hospital beds or specialists—those who do not merge may find themselves in an untenable market position. If large integrated organizations can supply all of the beds needed by the managed care market, who needs a stand-alone hospital? If these IDNs have contracts that cover specialty services, why would they refer patients outside the system? As a market integrates, many of the smaller players shop for the best deal they can find.

In the early stages of integration there is also intense competition for scarce resources—which almost always include primary care physicians. In most markets, primary care physicians are the entry point into the health care system and thus the source of patients, so the integrating networks vie to build alliances with or purchase the practices of primary care physicians. Other competition occurs for profitable suburban hospitals; for well-respected, well-managed group practices; and for pediatric or other specialty hospitals. All of this competition for partners quickly transforms any question of "Should we integrate?" to "With whom will we integrate?"

Fad or Fundamental Change?

The mergers that create today's IDNs are apt to be horizontal (multiple hospitals or multiple specialty practices) and vertical (involving at least hospitals and physician practices) simultaneously. Most feel that the combination of vertical and horizontal integration that characterizes today's integrating delivery networks is a durable concept based on four principles:

- Pressure on costs of health care will continue, and IDNs can provide care at a lower cost.
- IDNs can provide better customer service.
- Health care is a local business.
- Bigger is better when contracting with managed care organizations.

Opportunities to Reduce Costs

The first principle is not debated. We all recognize that technology advances will allow us to do more, but the pressure to make health care affordable will remain. We want to contain costs, but how will that be accomplished? At the most basic level, it will be through lowering the cost of inputs: supplies, pharmaceuticals, and staff levels. At the next level, money can be saved by eliminating duplicate tests and other unnecessary services or by consolidating services to gain operational economies of scale. A good way to save is through more efficient use of staff—the biggest ticket item in any health care organization's budget. As an example, Sharp Healthcare System developed an IDN-wide staffing process that permits available, qualified staff in one facility to fill needs in any other facility. The resulting first-year savings was $3.6 million dollars, mainly due to reduced overtime and reduced use of agency staff.[1]

The largest cost savings will come from delivering the right services at the right time in the right setting by making sure that effective preventive care is provided to all who can benefit, that errors in care are avoided, and that the most cost-effective approach to care is taken. Savings in supplies can be achieved though vertical integration or through buying cooperatives. Savings in care delivery, however, require that health services be coordinated, that incentives among providers be aligned, and that clear communication occurs among the providers of care and between providers and patients. IDNs can share the cost of investment in development and implementation of clinical protocols, they can fund staff to analyze practice patterns, and they can share the cost of investment in information systems to support cross-continuum communication.

Improved Customer Service

Customer service has become a new basis for competition in the health care marketplace. How can we make it easy for patients to access care, to obtain tools to improve self-care and informed decision making, to understand their bills, and to skip the unnecessary administrative tasks? Integration can provide the infrastructure and the organization to measure and improve customer service—sharing information efficiently is at least possible within one delivery system. The fact that a system is integrated also raises customers' expectations for service and continuity, while at the same time making good service and continuity of care challenging. Investments in customer services such as advice nurses and twenty-four-hour triage; centralized, coordinated appointment scheduling; and Web-based patient education are much more feasible if the dollars and skills required are pooled across multiple entities.

Keeping Health Care Local

Although some economies of scale can best be accomplished through achieving national (or even international) scale, health care is and likely will remain a local business. Patients seek care locally and referrals are to local providers. This means that to achieve optimal efficiency the services offered, hours of service, and even marketing should be tailored to local needs. This heavy local orientation obviates some of the advantages of chain businesses that are found in other industries.

Becoming Indispensable to Managed Care Organizations

Because many patients are now part of managed care systems, IDNs need to gain contracts with all (or at least most) of the large managed care organizations in their market. This requires that they be able to provide access across a wide geographical area (a requirement for patient convenience), which in turn requires a primary care network across the same territory. A combination of horizontal and vertical integration is essential to being an indispensable partner to managed care organizations.

For these and many other reasons, most observers feel that IDNs are a durable trend and will have many opportunities to add value to our health care system.

Critical Success Factors

The market has not yet developed to the point that anyone can define the rules that will guarantee successful integration. There is emerging consensus, however, that integration of physicians is one of the universal challenges, and integration between care delivery and financing seems to be one of the continuing questions.

In one 1996 survey, the CEOs of existing IDNs cited the most difficult challenges in building IDNs as aligning the organization with physicians, changing managers' mind-sets from a hospital to a system orientation, and creating effective governance structures.[2]

Dean Coddington, the principal researcher of a major study of integration published in 1996,[3] commented that integration was generally proceeding as predicted: by developing primary care networks, implementing clinical guidelines and clinical information systems, and expanding health plans (if part of the IDN). He cited purchasing primary care practices and integrating with a health plan as two problem areas. Acquiring primary care practices is capital-intensive and requires careful attention to productivity incentives to make them economically attractive. He also noted that the growth of "single-disease" providers (for example, cardiac, cancer, or orthopedic centers) and physician practice management companies may have an impact on the future course of integration.[4]

In a 1997 survey, 90 percent of health care system executives rated physician integration as critical to a system's success.[5] In the same survey, executives were asked to rate the success of different organizational structures for achieving that integration. The results indicate that most current organizational models leave a lot to be desired. For example, 75 percent of the executives reported that they have a management services organization for physicians, but only 11 percent rated the arrangement as effective; 51 percent have an open physician-hospital organization (PHO), and 19 percent rated it as effective; and 28 percent enlisted the physicians as joint owners of the managed care plan, but only 8 percent found this to be effective. Direct employment of physicians was reported to be the most effective means of ensuring integration; 74 percent reported using this arrangement, and 44 percent rated it as effective. This, however, was also the model cited as being the least profitable.

Some industry observers insist that the future is in integrated financing and delivery networks (IFDNs), but some of the most problematic mergers have come from trying to integrate financing and delivery. The breakup of Humana was an early, large-scale example of the disintegration of financing and delivery. Some mergers that are announced dissolve before they are completed (for example, Barnes Jewish Christian Health System and Missouri Blue Cross).

The most common reasons given for failure of mergers between financing and delivery are that the union is between two parties that formerly regarded themselves as enemies, and that the parties have conflicting incentives and expectations. Doctors want access to the latest technology; health plans want to reduce capital expenditures. A new treatment discovery is a cause for celebration and a marketing opportunity for a hospital, yet it causes concern about adverse selection among heath plan executives. Bill McNulty, an executive from Allina (one of the successful IFDNs), points out that what a health plan refers to as the medical loss ratio represents the reimbursement for the provider's clinical expertise and hard work.[6]

One Blue Cross executive summarized the difference between providers' and payers' perspectives on pricing service in an IFDN this way: "Providers at the table say, 'We are related, you should pay me more,' while the health plan staff argue, 'We are related, you should give me the best price.'"[6]

Physician practice management companies (PPMs) are seen by some as a threat to IDNs. Some of the more interesting PPMs (at least to Wall Street) are disease or specialty focused. By concentrating on, or "carving out," one practice area (typically specialties such as cardiology, oncology, or orthopedics, or diseases such as congestive heart failure), these organizations can develop deep expertise and detailed protocols for care. They can also acquire the most advanced equipment and create specialty treatment centers (sometimes financed through public offerings).

Though successful in negotiating carve-out arrangements with managed care plans, some of the earliest PPMs ran into trouble on the business side—managing finances, managing the practice, and so on.[7] These issues are correctable. The more important questions are, How do you achieve continuity of care if patients are treated in specialized centers? What happens if a cancer patient also has asthma? Are records duplicated in multiple locations? and How will clinical information flow from the carve-out providers to the other practitioners involved in a patient's care? The concept of PPMs appears to be aligned with treating disease but not with treating patients. Many hope that the future trend of patient care will be toward increasing integration, not toward more fragmentation (under any name).

Industry watcher Peter Boland has made an important bottom-line observation: consumers and payers do not care about the structure of an IDN—they care about performance. Our current health care systems will continue to be reshaped until they deliver better care at lower costs.[8] Later chapters of this book discuss some of the major reshaping efforts that are under way.

Measuring Integration

When we began to collaborate with IDNs on research projects (on issues related to new models of care and requirements for information support), we immediately ran into the problem of how to measure integration:

- What processes should be included in the measure? (For example, should we include processes related to marketing the health plan?)
- Should we use terms such as *clinical triage* or should we call the process *demand management?* Is there a difference?
- How can we identify organizations that are at similar stages of integration and that might be facing similar issues?
- How can we track progress and identify areas where there seem to be barriers to integration?
- How much integration is enough?

We realized that if we could develop measures of integration, they would improve communication within and among the integrating organizations—the information systems departments, the physicians, and the executive team all working on one vision of integration, building support for one set of processes, and aligning around one agenda for change. We began the process by asking the collaborating IDNs to discuss the fundamental differences between integrated and traditional delivery systems; this provided a basis for determining what to measure.

The next step was to review the literature on integration and try to extract a comprehensive set of attributes that would define integration. In the literature, we found several attempts to develop measures of integration, but some seemed too subjective to be applied consistently, too limited to measure all of the important aspects of integration, or too quantitative to be practical. Most also left out any measures of information integration, which all the collaborators agreed was a key enabler of clinical and operational integration. The review of past attempts to measure integration, however, did provide some ideas of both what to emulate and what to avoid.

One existing measure of integration is the "St. Anthony's system." It is used to rank IDNs on a scale of integration from 1 (low) to 5 (high) called "the five degrees of integration." The distinctions between the levels are subtle. For example, level-4 integration is defined as, "Provide a full range of care via several different types of providers. Many administrative functions, including purchasing, are centralized." Level 5 is defined as, "Provide a full range of care. Most administrative functions are performed for the entire system, typically by an even larger parent."[9]

In Shortell's study of nine delivery systems,[10] four dimensions of integration were identified:

- System culture/systemness: degree of commitment to a common culture and mission, reflected in the extent of coordination and joint value received from strategic, financial, and human resources planning and so on
- Physician–system integration: extent to which physicians benefit economically, are committed to using the system, and are involved with system administration
- Managed care: integration of financing with delivery for covered patients
- Clinical integration: the extent to which patient care services are coordinated among entities

Shortell rated organizations on more than one hundred dimensions of integration. For example, do operating units follow system compensation policies? Is at least one physician on the system board? How many physicians see more than fifty patients per year in settings owned by the system?

A comprehensive study of integrated delivery for the Center for Research in Ambulatory Health Care Administration[3] identified several common attributes of mature IDNs:

Physicians play a key leadership role.

The organization's structure promotes coordination.

Primary care providers are economically integrated.

Practice sites provide geographic coverage.

Resources are balanced with demand.

Physicians are organized.

Health plans are owned or are partners.

Financial incentives are aligned.

Clinical and management information systems tie system elements together, and the system has access to financial resources and the ability to shift them.

After reviewing these three and other integration measures, we decided to create a new set of measures that would be as explicit as possible (leaving little room for interpretation), available (no extensive data collection and analysis required), and encompassing (all key aspects of integration included). What has evolved (and will continue to evolve over time) is the Scottsdale Institute/First Consulting Group Integration Index. The index comprises a series of thirty-three attributes, all of which are assessed on a four-point scale: none, just beginning to integrate across settings, somewhat there, or totally integrated. This is a classification system, not a grading mechanism—a high score means that there is more integration, not necessarily that there is better integration (because there are no data to indicate what level and type of integration is enough).

The Integration Index is segmented into four dimensions of integration: structural, operational, clinical, and informational. (The first three are found in several other scoring systems; information integration was added because it is a critical enabler of the operational and clinical processes).

Structural integration refers to the initial legal and organizational integration. As one CEO put it, "this is when the lawyers and sign painters get paid." The attributes of structural integration include offering primary, specialist, and hospital care; operating a health plan; having a single CEO and board; having one corporate mission statement, one business strategy, and one organizational chart; and defining management jobs, performance measures, and incentives in terms of the IDN's business objectives.

Operational integration includes redefining and redesigning the business processes of the new enterprise to achieve operational efficiencies. Measures of operational integration include having common corporate processes; having functions, budgets, and financial statements that are organized around corporate programs rather than individual care settings; and using one peer review and credentialing process.

Clinical integration is the ultimate goal of many integration efforts. Measures of clinical integration include providing access to care throughout the enterprise in a coordinated manner, being able to track outcomes of care episodes across settings, and maintaining wellness as an active part of the delivery system.

Information integration measures the extent to which the new enterprise has the information infrastructure, communications, and applications to support operational and clinical integration. The attributes include the abilities to identify each member or patient across care settings, to update patient clinical and administrative information once and make it available to all authorized users, to maintain one integrated patient problem list, to coordinate the scheduling of visits across settings, to enable care providers to communicate seamlessly across settings, and to analyze outcomes of care across settings.

We translated these attributes into a survey format and, in early 1996, assessed the level of integration on these four dimensions. The initial participants were executives of IDNs that were members of the Center for Clinical Integration (now the Scottsdale Institute). A total of forty organizations participated in the initial survey (an 80 percent response rate). The respondents include many of the organizations that are cited as leaders in the integration trend.

How Integrated Are We?

The results of our initial survey were revealing. The highest scores were for attributes of structural integration. As shown in Figure 1.1, only one organization reported that it was in the beginning stages of structural integration, and eleven appear to be in the home stretch toward achieving total integration on the structural attributes we identified.

FIGURE 1.1. INTEGRATION SURVEY RESULTS.

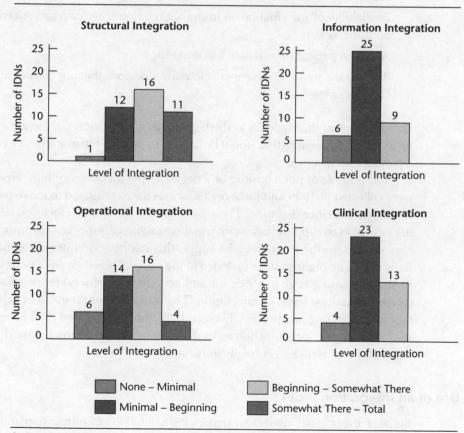

A few organizations reported significant progress on aspects of operational integration, and one-half of the group had crossed the line between "beginning" to "somewhat there." The picture shifts, however, when we look at clinical integration, for which no organization had aggregate scores in the highest category ("somewhat there" to "totally integrated"), but the majority were beginning to make progress. The lowest aggregate scores were in the area of information integration. The IDNs in this group did not yet have the information infrastructure in place to achieve high levels of integration from the patient care perspective.

An analysis of the individual attributes was revealing as well. The areas where the least progress had been made were all related to information integration:

Integrated patient problem list

Information on patients' primary care providers

Ability of providers to communicate seamlessly across settings

Availability of information on insurance requirements (coverage, need for authorizations)

Access to patient information across settings

Tools at the point of service to help make decisions that are consistent with "best practices"

Looking back at the vignettes at the beginning of this chapter, these are exactly the types of capabilities that would be needed to provide integrated services from a patient's perspective.

It is possible to put a positive or a negative spin on these findings. First, they were collected in 1996 and these organizations have continued to make progress on integration since that time. There has been a major market focus on developing new tools to support patient information exchange, especially in ambulatory care settings, so the technology for supporting information integration has also improved. The organizations included in the sample, however, were perceived to be on the leading edge in 1996; it is unlikely that the general market has even caught up to these levels of integration. The other factor to remember is that integration is an ongoing process. Even an IDN that has achieved total integration may add another organization to its delivery network, in which case the next day the system is no longer totally integrated.

Use of an Integration Index

Some of the original motives for developing a definition of integration and an integration index were discussed earlier. Once we developed the tool, we found additional uses. One is to provide a common baseline for planning. In a few of the original participating organizations, we obtained multiple assessments from different executives at the same organization. The assessments were generally consistent, except that CIOs tended to report lower levels of information integration than other executives. Because information systems are a key enabler of integration and because everyone agrees that "informating" the IDN is not an easy task, this may indicate that CEOs have underestimated some of the challenges ahead. Comparing ratings within an executive team is a good way to set realistic expectations of the work to be done.

Most integrating delivery organizations believe that they are behind the market and need to catch up. When we use the survey to compare the level of integration at a particular site with the consolidated database, we often find that the gap is not large. It is useful for organizations to know that although they may be far from where they want to be, they are not as far behind the market as they thought. The need for progress may be urgent, but it does not require a panic move.

As is discussed in later chapters, we also found that the level of integration is a way to define peer groups for comparison. Examining this level of operational integration helped explain the differences in capital investment levels in information systems that we found in our recent benchmarking study, discussed in Chapter Nine. The College of Healthcare Information Management Executives (CHIME) has included some of the integration attributes in its annual information management survey. This will allow CHIME to make a similar comparison.

In Appendix A we have included a copy of the integration measurement tool that was used to compile the data discussed in this chapter. (We have added and deleted several questions over the years, and some of the original questions have been moved to different categories.) Using this tool to perform a self-assessment, readers can compare their level of integration with the original forty IDNs in our study.

One of the conclusions of Coddington's study of nine successful IDNs sums up current mainstream thinking on IDNs: "The key to an integrated delivery system is not what form it takes, but what difference it makes. To justify its existence and the acceptance of change required by everyone involved, an integrated system must add value for its patients and purchasers, improve the competitive position of its sponsors, and satisfy the needs of its physicians and hospitals. It takes talented people to meet these objectives."[3]

We believe that to deliver performance, IDNs must radically redesign core processes across the continuum and make significant investments in information systems. In the chapters that follow we relate some early experiences with making these fundamental changes in health care delivery.

Notes

1. Davis, A. "Managing Staff Resources Through Automation." *ADVANCE*, June 1997, pp. 53–55.
2. Greene, J. "Integrated Delivery Looms as Most Significant Issue for System Executives." *Modern Healthcare*, Aug. 5, 1996, pp. 91–94.
3. Coddington, D. C., Moore, K. D., and Fischer, E. A. *Making Integrated Health Care Work*. Englewood, Colo.: Center for Research in Ambulatory Health Care Administration, 1996.
4. Anonymous. "Evaluating Integrated Healthcare Trends: An Interview with Dean Coddington." *Healthcare Financial Management*, Sept. 1997, pp. 40–42.
5. Japsen, B. "The Reluctant Doctor: Survey Finds Luring Physicians into Systems Is Tough." *Modern Healthcare*, 1997, *27*, 66–68.
6. Bilchik, G. S. "Can Rivals Play Nice?" *Hospitals and Health Networks*, Apr. 20, 1997, pp. 24–28.
7. Cochrane, J. D. "PPM Growth Strategies." *Integrated Healthcare Report*, July 1997, pp. 1–10.
8. Anonymous. "Look at It This Way." *Hospitals and Health Networks*, 1996, *70*, 66–76.
9. Solovy, A. "The Health Care 100." *Hospitals and Health Networks*, Mar. 20, 1997, pp. 35–49.
10. Shortell, S. M., and others. *Remaking Health Care in America*. San Francisco: Jossey-Bass, 1996.

CHAPTER TWO

A PROCESS FRAMEWORK FOR THE INTEGRATED DELIVERY NETWORK OF THE 21STCENTURY

Erica Drazen and Jane Metzger

As integrating delivery networks build new enterprise processes, they all respond to similar business pressures and face the challenge of transforming similarly fragmented legacy organizations and processes. Most have comparable visions of the ideal future integrated system of care and improved health status of the population. They work hard on integration, and all make massive investments in changing processes and implementing information technology. Many also share a desire to find organizations from whom they can gain insights about critical success factors in achieving their visions and with whom they can discuss common problems and perhaps jointly fund solutions.

We formed a collaborative with five integrating delivery networks that were members of the Scottsdale Institute. These organizations wanted to share their experiences and the lessons they had learned about major process redesign and effective information support. As a group, we quickly made three observations:

- Although the organizations had a similar vision of the future, the path to achieve that vision was unclear.
- There was concern among all participants that without clarity about the path, many of the investments being made today might not be durable building blocks for the future.
- Communication was hampered by the lack of consistent terminology among the group—participants used terms such as *access to care, care management,* and *medical management* to mean quite different things.

To provide a framework for discussion and collaboration, we identified the principles that will define the future state of integrated care and then built a high-level process framework for that future. This allowed us to position the activities under way today within the context of a future process. For example, patient scheduling has traditionally been seen as part of "practice management." Computer systems purchased to support scheduling are often part of a system that provides both scheduling and billing support. In the future framework, however, patient scheduling is part of the process of engaging and retaining members, with close ties to enrollment and care management. This is a very different process with a distinct set of information requirements.

The process framework is a taxonomy that helps ensure that we are defining processes that will meet the future goals of our IDNs. This framework does not define the details of how the actual process will be accomplished—process steps, participants, locations, timing, patient and data flows, and so forth. For instance, new access to care approaches incorporate elements of the processes related to engaging members, assessing health status, and delivering care. These are found in different parts of the framework rather than in a typical sequence. The framework does, however, contain all of the activities we found in emerging process models. We have found that taking this decomposed view of the building blocks of the future delivery process is useful in understanding the new elements of future models and getting an early look at the information management challenges they represent.

As discussed in Chapter One, IDNs are working simultaneously on many patient care and business processes. In our research we decided to focus initially on the processes of care delivery. Of course the successful integrated care system will also require lean and effective administrative business processes. The care processes, however, represent the core health business of the IDN. The current options for the care process are more open ended than, for example, the choices for business processes such as financial or human resource management. There is also great uncertainty about how to integrate and coordinate across the continuum of care.

The Process Framework

Our goal was to understand and help transfer knowledge about design, implementation, and support of care delivery processes that would create the future IDN. We first identified the overarching principles for the future and developed an overall process framework for organizing new process activities. For patient care, this includes the five top-level processes shown in Figure 2.1. We then defined underlying subprocesses and activities for each top-level process. This resulted in the four-level process hierarchy illustrated in Figure 2.2.

FIGURE 2.1. TOP-LEVEL PROCESSES
OF THE FUTURE IDN PROCESS FRAMEWORK.

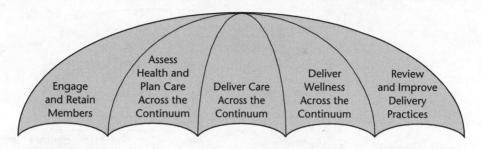

The framework was developed and refined iteratively, and we expect it to remain a work in progress for some time. We initially sought information from the following internal and external sources:

- "Visions of the future" statements and descriptions from information technology strategic plans
- Documents on redesign that describe operational principles and process flows for care management
- Information system requirements specified for new enterprise processes (which include many hints about how processes enabled by information technology are expected to work)
- Descriptions of process innovations in trade magazines and research publications

A preliminary draft of the framework was reviewed by our associates who work with leading IDNs in engagements relating to new integrated care processes and by the IDNs that participated in the collaborative. As a final step in the process, we identified performance metrics that could be used to measure progress toward the ultimate goals of clinical and operational integration.

Once the overall framework was in place, we identified two umbrella processes for closer study: engage and retain members, and assess health and plan care across the continuum. These processes were chosen because they were the focus of re-design efforts in several of the collaborating IDNs. Working with the collaborating organizations, we identified sites that had experience in redesigning these areas and conducted site visits and interviews to learn more about the redesign efforts, the benefits they had realized, and the critical success factors involved. We then brought this information to the collaborators' teams. These activities provided a

FIGURE 2.2. FOUR LEVELS OF THE
PROCESS FRAMEWORK FOR THE FUTURE IDN.

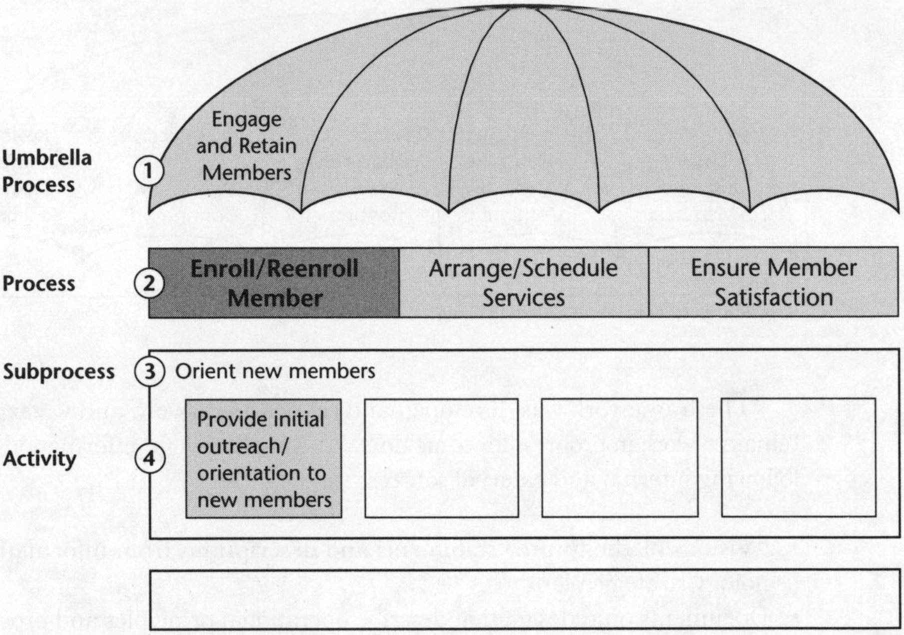

Umbrella Process (1)	Engage and Retain Members	

Process (2)	**Enroll/Reenroll Member**	Arrange/Schedule Services	Ensure Member Satisfaction

Subprocess (3)	Orient new members			
Activity (4)	Provide initial outreach/ orientation to new members			

detailed look at the care processes that are being developed and gave us an opportunity to discuss goals and approaches with staff involved in redesign efforts in several sites. We used the information we obtained to enhance and validate the initial process framework. We identified numerous new activities and subdivided and reorganized portions of the framework. Figures 2.3 through 2.7 show the detailed subprocess charts for the two umbrella processes we validated in this way.

These umbrella processes include the activities that are involved in organizing patient connections and communication with the health care system and in care management. As we proceeded with our research on these two processes, we discovered that they are also the first enterprise care processes that are being implemented by IDNs. The subprocesses of arranging and scheduling services (Figure 2.4) are the sources of greatest consumer dissatisfaction and are being redesigned to improve member satisfaction and retention. The health assessment and planning processes (Figures 2.6 and 2.7) are where organizations feel they can

FIGURE 2.3. ENROLL/REENROLL MEMBER.

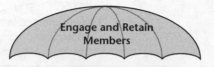

Enroll/Reenroll Member	Arrange/Schedule Services	Ensure Member Satisfaction

Set standards and monitor performance

Develop and adopt service enrollment and encounter standards	Document member preferences regarding enrollment	Educate members concerning enrollment and encounter standards	Monitor performance of enrollment processes	Market customer service and quality standards to patients and prospective patients

Obtain and retain members

Identify new members	Enroll, reenroll, or disenroll member	Perform/Update registration	Identify and follow up inactive members

Orient new members

Provide initial outreach/ orientation to new members	Profile member needs and preferences	Provide member or patient card, ID numbers, and orientation materials	Coach in PCP selection	Conduct initial risk screening of new members

Conduct preliminary member assessment and assignment to care model

Match new members with appropriate care delivery model	Assemble new member prior medical history	Connect members with relevant knowledge sources and support groups	Connect members with provider team	Reassess care model based on change in status/referrals

Maintain accuracy and awareness of contact information

Provide caregiver/team contact information to members	Verify/Update changes to member contact information	Notify caregivers of changes in member's eligibility/ coverage	Notify caregivers of changes to patient contact information	Notify caregivers of member PCP selection/ change

FIGURE 2.4. ARRANGE/SCHEDULE SERVICES.

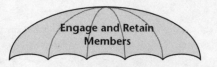

Enroll/Reenroll Member	**Arrange/Schedule Services**	Ensure Member Satisfaction

Set standards and monitor performance

Develop and adopt service access and encounter standards	Document member preferences regarding access	Educate members concerning service access and encounter standards	Monitor performance service access processes	Market customer service and quality standards to patients and prospective patients

Arrange services

Maintain schedules	Manage wait lists	Manage referrals

Book/rebook/cancel appointments	Triage patient requests for services	Accommodate member needs and preferences	Check compliance with protocols (locations, clinical appropriateness)

Manage patient accounts

Capture/update insurance information	Verify patient eligibility and coverage	Advise patient of financial implications of requested services

Advise patient of current account status	Provide financial counseling	Collect and post patient co-pays and other payments

Provide access-related patient information and education

Provide service instructions to patients with appointments	Provide confirmation/reminders to patients with appointments	Notify patients of appointment changes	Notify members to schedule needed follow-up and wellness services

Monitor service completion

Notify caregivers of patients with incomplete services	Notify caregivers of patients with overdue services	Follow-up patients with incomplete services	Follow-up patients with overdue services

Copyright © 1998 by First Consulting Group.

FIGURE 2.5. ENSURE MEMBER SATISFACTION.

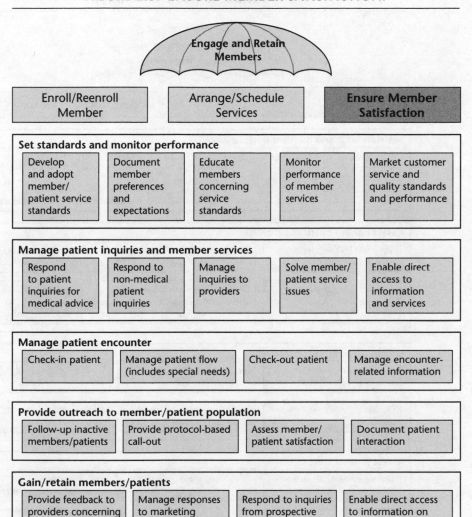

Engage and Retain Members

Enroll/Reenroll Member	Arrange/Schedule Services	**Ensure Member Satisfaction**

Set standards and monitor performance

Develop and adopt member/ patient service standards	Document member preferences and expectations	Educate members concerning service standards	Monitor performance of member services	Market customer service and quality standards and performance

Manage patient inquiries and member services

Respond to patient inquiries for medical advice	Respond to non-medical patient inquiries	Manage inquiries to providers	Solve member/ patient service issues	Enable direct access to information and services

Manage patient encounter

Check-in patient	Manage patient flow (includes special needs)	Check-out patient	Manage encounter-related information

Provide outreach to member/patient population

Follow-up inactive members/patients	Provide protocol-based call-out	Assess member/ patient satisfaction	Document patient interaction

Gain/retain members/patients

Provide feedback to providers concerning service issues	Manage responses to marketing campaigns	Respond to inquiries from prospective members	Enable direct access to information on resources and services

FIGURE 2.6. ASSESS HEALTH.

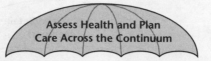

Assess Health and Plan
Care Across the Continuum

Assess Health	Develop Care and Wellness Plan

Set standards and monitor performance

Develop and adopt patient service standards	Document members' preferences and expectations	Educate members about service standards	Monitor performance	Market standards and performance

Assess patient health/health risks

Obtain relevant assessment tools for care model	Obtain and review health history	Identify hereditary and environmental risk factors
Assess lifestyle and self-management capability	Obtain patient compliance and socioeconomic risk factors	Obtain patient's self-assessment (functional status) and health needs

Follow-up progress proactively

Monitor compliance with care and wellness plans	Identify unplanned interventions	Verify completion of planned interventions
Obtain patient's self-monitoring results	Notify care team of patient progress	Obtain assessments of extended care team

Assess patient status

Obtain relevant assessment tools for care models	Diagnose illness	Perform specialty consultation upon referral
Monitor status of referrals for evaluation/treatment	Assess progress against treatment/wellness goals	Document assessment of patient condition/wellness

Empower patients

Educate patient regarding condition/health risk factors	Customize patient education materials	Document education and patient comprehension
Connect patient with relevant information resources	Enable direct access to self-assessment instruments and tools	Communicate all relevant information to patient

FIGURE 2.7. DEVELOP CARE AND WELLNESS PLAN.

Assess Health and Plan
Care Across the Continuum

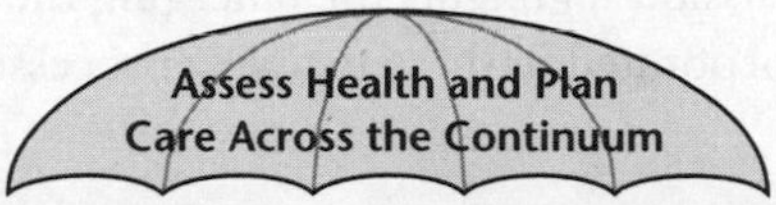

Assess Health	Develop Care and Wellness Plan

Set standards and monitor performance

Develop and adopt patient service standards	Document members' preferences and expectations	Educate members about service standards	Monitor performance	Market performance

Develop wellness plan

Obtain relevant protocols and guidelines	Establish goals for patient wellness	Address patient self-management profile/preferences
Schedule planned interventions	Develop/document wellness plan (goals, interventions)	Communicate relevant information to care team

Initiate wellness plan (activate protocols, order intervention) including follow-up

Develop care plan

Obtain relevant care management proto-cols and guidelines	Establish goals for patient recovery	Address patient self-management profile/preferences	Initiate care episode and engage care team
Develop/document care plan (goals, interventions)	Initiate care plan (activate protocols, order intervention) including follow-up	Schedule planned interventions	Communicate relevant information to care team

Engage and manage referrals

Identify need for referral	Ensure appropriateness of referral	Authorize/obtain authorization for referral
Identify and engage care team for referral	Engage external and community providers	Communicate relevant information to referral providers

Empower patient

Provide information on care management options	Collaborate in review of alternatives	Coach patient about self-care and obtaining follow-up care
Develop patient self-management contract	Document education and patient comprehension	Communicate relevant infor-mation to patient and family

Enable direct access to information resources on care and wellness create the greatest value in improved health status and reduced costs of care. The following discussion highlights the emerging themes and resulting activities that are being incorporated in these two new processes.

Themes Leading to New Activities

Several recurring themes can be observed in emerging models for patient care delivery and management. These are oriented toward realizing business objectives that make the new process seamless, customer friendly, proactive, cross-continuum, and integrated.

Reaching Out to Patients as Partners

Traditional ways of organizing health care have put most of the burden for initiating a care transaction on the patient, and the job of responding in the hands of the health care system. Commonplace examples include waiting for the first contact from a newly enrolled patient, responding to requests for services, and relying on a patient to telephone for results of diagnostic tests or procedures.

In both of the emerging processes examined in our research, there is a conscious effort to reverse the traditional roles in some situations. Outreach is important in establishing a partnership in care and in anticipating and managing care needs in a more timely and reliable way. Examples of outreach include calling to check on patients who have received telephone advice, sending reminders about overdue preventive services, and conducting initial health assessments at a member's work site as part of the managed care enrollment process. Accomplishing outreach requires new supporting roles to organize and perform the work and new mechanisms for tracking patients and following up with them. Outreach also introduces new activities such as making initial contact and providing orientation to new members, as well as following up with inactive members (Figure 2.3).

Empowering Patients in Self-Management

Patients control everything about their health care status and recovery except the direct care interventions delivered by the care system. New models seek to empower patients to be effective in self-management through access to education, information, resources, and support. Formalizing patient responsibility and increasing patient skill and knowledge to enable them to assume the responsibility are widely viewed as cost-effective investments and appropriate roles of a health care system. Much attention is being paid to gaining a better understanding of patient lifestyles and options for care and then sharing that understanding with patients and family members. New activities to empower patients include connecting them with relevant information resources (Figure 2.6) and developing patient self-management contracts (Figure 2.7). The net effect is the sharing of both knowledge and decision-making responsibility. In some cases technology is providing new ways to support these goals (for example, enabling access to patient education materials through a Web site).

Supporting Patients in Doing the Right Thing

There are at least four elements to supporting patients in their efforts to seek care appropriately and maintain their health status:

- Making sure that patients know (and agree with) what they should do
- Making sure they know how to do the right thing
- Making it easy (or as easy as possible) to comply
- Providing reminders and other supports that increase the likelihood of success

New models incorporate many activities that support one or several of these elements, including ensuring that all relevant information is communicated to patients (Figure 2.6), collaborating with patients in determining their care strategy (Figure 2.7), and coaching patients about self-care and obtaining follow-up care (Figure 2.7).

IDNs are already combining these activities in innovative ways. For example, one site uses electronic medical records systems to provide patients with reports on their visits to the doctor, including patient education materials that have been tailored to address patients' specific problems and follow-up treatment requirements. The research supporting this innovation showed that

- Patients have a hard time "hearing" all of a physician's instructions when they are at the doctor's office.
- Patients are likely to have questions when they return home.
- Information that is endorsed by a physician and tailored to a patient's needs is viewed as having much greater value than generic preprinted brochures.[1]

Focusing on the Customer

Taking the patient's view of the care process is a core principle in current redesign efforts. This is the only way to craft a care relationship with the patient and an experience for the customer that is understandable, easy to navigate, and effective.

This theme is leading to substantial centralization and integration of customer access points for obtaining services and information. Principles and operational models from other service industries are increasingly being adopted in health care. A good example is the telephone access center, where patients can schedule an appointment, receive medical triage and advice, change their primary care physician designation, or sign up for a patient education class.

The care experience is being redesigned so that providers in different disciplines, sites, and settings can function as part of a coordinated system. Integrated care leads to new activities that focus expressly on coordination so that patients no longer must navigate on their own. Some new activities, such as communicating relevant information on patient progress to the care team (Figure 2.6), focus on transferring information to coordinate care. Other activities, such as connecting new members with their provider team (Figure 2.3), accomplish coordination more directly. Customer focus also means that more attention is paid to customer convenience and preference. This requires both capturing the information (profiling member needs and preferences, Figure 2.3) and incorporating preferences in arranging services (Figure 2.4) and in care plans (Figure 2.7).

Tailoring Care Management to Patient Needs

Doing a better job for each patient requires understanding not only health status but also self-management capacity, communication style, and health-care-seeking behavior. Traditionally physicians have flagged certain patients for more proactive follow-up (put some patients on a "watch list") and over time have come to understand how best to communicate with, motivate, and support patients. New models attempt to accomplish this in a more coordinated and systematic way by tailoring both the process for care management and the clinical management approach to match the needs of similar subgroups of patients. For example, patients with chronic disease who are expected to use many health services may be served in a designated ambulatory center and assigned to a case manager who works with a physician and other providers to ensure that care is delivered as planned. Accomplishing this requires new activities such as matching and connecting each patient with the appropriate care model and provider team (Figure 2.3). The process of accessing care can also be tailored to fit the needs and expectations of different groups of patients. Some patients might benefit from a work-site clinic, whereas on-site triage in a community health center would be better for others; communication by Web access for those conversant in Internet technology would be ideal, whereas telephone contact would be more helpful for others.

Supporting Providers in Doing the Right Thing

Many of the business objectives for a new care delivery process relate to ensuring that patients receive a consistent standard of care, independent of the location where that care is provided. For individual patients this means they receive appropriate care and support based on the current understanding of good clinical practice. A process for developing consensus of best practices is being defined in most IDNs. The more advanced sites are also experimenting with different approaches to deploying best practices. The goal is to have information on relevant good practices available each time a patient management decision is made.

Additional activities are being incorporated to support providers in keeping track of the patients they do not see, ensuring that follow-up care occurs, and staying abreast of their patients' progress. Many activities focus on consistent capture of information that will aid providers in doing the right thing; others focus on proactive notification concerning planned and unplanned occurrences and clinical findings needed by providers. Many of these activities are geared to closing process or communication loops that can result in delays and oversights. For example, closing loops requires proactive activities such as verifying the completion of planned interventions (Figure 2.6) and following up with patients with incomplete services (Figure 2.4).

Turning Handoffs into Seamless Transitions

Traditional care processes are replete with handoffs between caregivers, departments, and sites and settings of care. Despite best efforts to the contrary, every handoff represents an opportunity for delays, for rework due to incomplete information accompanying the transfer of responsibility, and for potential errors of omission or commission. New activities are geared to expanding job roles to reduce handoffs and increase the coordination of care to ensure task completion, as well as to provide proactive information management to make any remaining handoffs seamless for both patients and caregivers (for example, to communicate relevant information to referral providers, Figure 2.7).

Understanding and Improving Practice

Implicit in the desire to provide appropriate care management for each patient is the need to understand and continually improve care practices and processes. Activities that are being incorporated into care management will capture the information necessary to examine practices. Providing an information base for practice analysis will require more information that is more structured and consistently recorded than the information that is being captured today. Accomplishing the multiple goals for new processes that depend on this information will require efficient procedures and tools if capturing information as a by-product of the care process is to be feasible.

Uses of the Process Framework

These themes resulted in the subprocesses and activities that appear in the process framework. The original intent of the process framework was twofold: to establish a lexicon for communication among the collaborating IDNs and to help put today's integration initiatives in the context of the IDN of the 21st Century. We also found that the framework provided an effective vehicle for sharing knowledge. As we learned about new approaches to process design, new performance metrics, and new benefits, we defined a structure in which to store that knowledge so that it could be retrieved and used in the future.

During the collaborative research process, we became more and more convinced that a process framework (rather than an organizational chart) was the only effective way to plan for integration; processes are what integrate an organization.

After the initial research project was completed, we began to incorporate this process framework into an approach to strategic information management planning. After the business strategies of an IDN are defined, we identify the processes that will be key to achieving the strategies. Next, information requirements are defined that support those key processes. The performance metrics we defined in the research project are a starter set for defining measures of success. We have found that use of a process framework helps liberate old mind-sets and also decreases the tendency to defend established organizational boundaries. Because this process framework is future-focused, organizations are pulled toward new models of care and challenged to think, for instance, about whether a traditional patient-scheduling process will serve them well. Perhaps they really should reevaluate the entire process of arranging services, which could include verifying eligibility, managing referrals, and reminding patients of preventive services that are due.

The process framework is also useful in process redesign. Not all activities are relevant to every IDN today. For example, an organization may be rethinking the front end of its care system but not yet working on care management. Reviewing likely future additions aids in designing a process (and information support) that accommodates the future and helps stage the migration to the future model.

From Framework to Process

Figure 2.8 depicts the major determinants of new enterprise processes at a high level. The current business drivers for strategic change in health care are consistent, although the pace varies in different markets. Each health care system translates these drivers into specific business objectives for new enterprise processes based on the role and definition of change in the organization's business strategy. For example, for some systems, being a community-focused and friendly provider may be the strategic direction and the area in which they invest the most change. For others, the goal may be to stay abreast of community standards for customer service and to focus elsewhere (such as on recognition as a center of clinical excellence) for differentiation. Strategies such as these define the business objectives that guide how new patient-care processes take shape.

The activities in the process framework become patient care delivery processes only when they are organized into actual staff roles and a multitude of decisions are made about steps that will be taken to accomplish the activity—triggers, sequencing, timing, location, information flows, and so forth. As an organization begins this task, the activities in the framework are like a deck of cards that can be sorted into different sets and combinations. Implementing new enterprise processes also requires attention to organization (governance, policies, and procedures) and to information management.

Chapters Three through Eight examine these issues by exploring emerging models for two new enterprise patient care delivery processes: *access to care*—the front end of care delivery and management (Chapters Three, Four, and Five); and *cross-continuum care management*—first manifested in new care models for patients

FIGURE 2.8. MAJOR DETERMINANTS OF NEW ENTERPRISE PROCESSES.

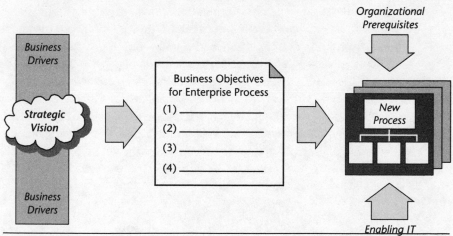

with chronic disease (Chapters Six, Seven, and Eight). For each process, the first chapter in the set (Chapters Three and Six, respectively) reviews the spectrum of process models in terms of scope and centralized coordination and the initial experience with organizational challenges. The following chapters (Chapters Four and Seven, respectively) discuss information management requirements for each process. To illustrate the new processes in action, the final chapter in each set (Chapters Five and Eight) provides a scenario-based view of the routine workday for key health care system players and the patient.

Notes

1. Tang, P. C., Newcomb, C., Gorden, S., and Kreider, N. "Meeting the Information Needs of Patients: Results from a Patient Focus Group." In D. R. Masys (ed.), *Journal of the American Medical Informatics Association Fall Proceedings*, 1997, pp. 672–676.

CHAPTER THREE

ACCESS TO CARE: NEW MODELS

Jane Metzger, Marty Geisler, and Sharon Graugnard

Scheduling and other processes for gaining access to health care services are among the first targets (if not the first) for redesign in integrating health care networks.

In a recent survey, chief information officers (CIOs) summarized the level of activity in one key process, enterprise scheduling, as follows: 12 percent had rolled out systemwide appointment and resource scheduling, 63 percent were in some stage of implementation, 23 percent had planned but not started implementation, and only 2 percent were not contemplating implementation.[1]

A recent survey of CIOs by the College of Healthcare Information Management Executives (CHIME) posed a different question, but the response also substantiates the emphasis on the front end of the care system: one of the top three current information technology priorities for CIOs was enterprise scheduling.[2]

This chapter reviews the reasons that health care providers focus on the access process. It also describes the emerging models, based on the pattern revealed by analyzing numerous case examples.

Because so many organizations are in some stage of implementing new models, we did not have to rely on visions and plans to research the process. Identifying case examples, however, required a bit of detective work. There are no industry conferences on enterprise access processes and there is very little published information on the topic. A literature search did yield descriptions of new models in a number of organizations and helped us identify others that we could investigate by telephone. We especially targeted project staff in sites with aggressive models (in terms of the degree of change from traditional access processes) or significant implementation experience for telephone follow-up and, in some cases, site visits.

Another major source was the ongoing redesign and piloting of new access models among our research collaborators within the Scottsdale Institute (then known as the Center for Clinical Integration). In discussions with their project staff, we learned a great deal about their business objectives and about many of the trade-offs they encountered in design and implementation. We also identified many case examples from our field experience, assembled available documents, and interviewed project staff to obtain more details.

We interviewed staff from four vendor organizations that provide triage services or software. Triage and medical advice is a major new component of the access process in many sites. These interviews gave us an opportunity to understand the service providers' perspective on the goals of health care organizations and other sponsors of triage and medical advice, as well as insight into how they structure and implement the process.

Two relevant industry collaborations were identified. Although they did not explicitly address enterprisewide access, publications and conferences resulting from the collaborations provided a view of the objectives and results of a more local focus on the access process. The first of these collaborations—by the HMO Group—was a benchmarking review of health plans with exemplary practices in appointment scheduling.[3] The second was a conference and publication resulting from a collaboration organized by the Institute for Healthcare Improvement to address unnecessary waits and delays in the provision of health care.[4,5] Both of these collaborations illustrate the complexity of portions of the access process and what it takes to make them function efficiently and consistently.

Collectively these sources provided many case examples and a wealth of information on emerging models that is discussed in this chapter. Specific health care organizations are named only when the information has been released in a publication; we adopted this practice to respect client confidentiality and our agreements with our research collaborators.

The chapter reviews the traditional access processes that health care organizations and networks are transforming and discusses the business drivers for change. Emerging process models are described and organized into three categories that represent increasing levels of change. We review the many organizational challenges presented by the new process models, as well as experience accumulated to date in overcoming these challenges. The final section of the chapter presents conclusions from the research and predictions for the future.

The Starting Point: Traditional Access Processes

Traditional processes by which patients access services have evolved over time, more to meet the needs of each departmental service center than to provide better customer service. Patients are presented with numerous access points, each with unique and sometimes idiosyncratic procedures. The resulting process for accessing services within the settings and sites of an emerging enterprise is very much a maze for patients and family members who seek services or information, as shown in Figure 3.1.

Typically, patients can expect to make multiple telephone calls and repeat their insurance, address change, and other information many times. They are more than likely to find long waits until the next available appointment. When they arrive to receive care, they make numerous stops to register, present a payer card, and make co-payments and pay other charges. They also spend a lot of time (perhaps in different parts of their encounter and in multiple service locations) waiting to check in, to be seen, or to check out.

This myriad of local processes did not evolve according to some grand design. Rather, it is a natural consequence of local management and accountability for each departmental profit center and physician practice, and of the largely local billing processes and systems put in place to support each "business." The goal in every health care organization that is becoming an integrated system is to transform this legacy into a rational, customer-friendly, and efficient process.

Business Drivers of Change

Health care organizations are all responding to similar business pressures as they build new enterprise processes for access to care.

Competition and Customer Service

Improving access to care is a business priority for many health care organizations because of competition. The resulting shift from thinking of patients as *patients* to thinking of them as *customers* has brought into health care the concept of customer service, a well-established business practice in other service industries.

Patients consider access an important element of the service of health care. In one research study, patients rated the following aspects of access as important:[6]

Seeing the same physician all the time	61 percent
Being able to get an appointment quickly	48 percent
Going to a physician who spends enough time with the patient	44 percent

FIGURE 3.1. TYPICAL ACCESS MODEL AS IT APPEARS TO PATIENTS.

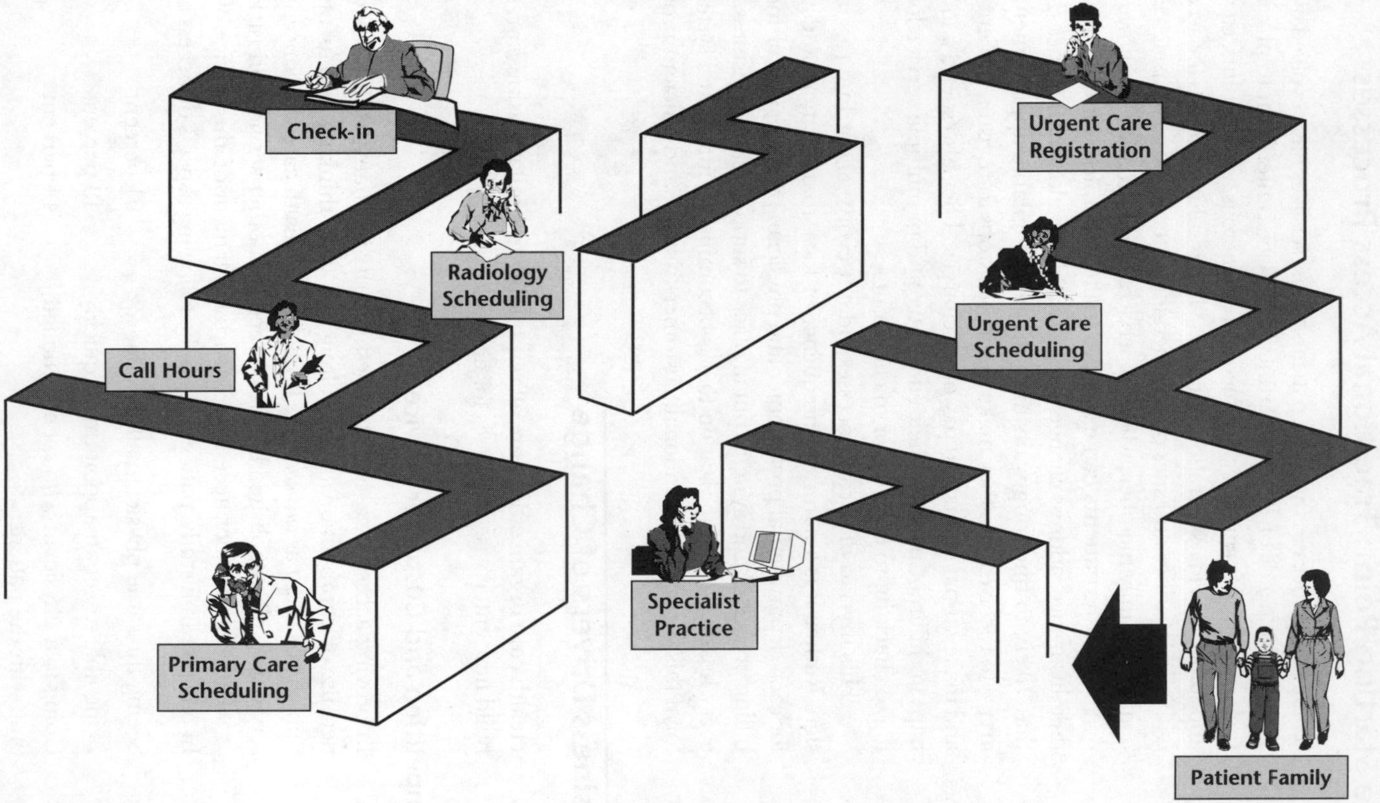

Urgent Care Registration

Urgent Care Scheduling

Patient Family

Specialist Practice

Check-in

Radiology Scheduling

Call Hours

Primary Care Scheduling

No long waits at the physician's office	34 percent
Convenient location	29 percent
Convenient hours	23 percent

Satisfaction with access also turns out to be a good predictor of overall patient satisfaction. Surveys of thirty thousand managed care patients showed that consumers who are satisfied with their routine care access are 4.8 times more likely to be satisfied with their health care service overall than those who are not.[7]

Each time patients access the system by telephone or in person, they have an array of tangible performance measures on which to judge the service they receive:

How many times and how many different locations they must call

How long they wait for the calls to be answered

Whether the service or information they need is available

How many times they have to check in

How many times they are asked to provide or verify the same information

How much time they spend during an encounter waiting for rather than receiving service

Traditional front-end processes fare poorly on all of these counts.

Health care organizations that study access are often shocked to learn that as many as one in five callers hangs up because it takes so long for their call to be answered. Lag times for urgent care appointments are often weeks; those for routine appointments are sometimes months.[4] One study of patient waiting times in a large outpatient clinic revealed an average total visit time of more than ninety-nine minutes, with nearly an hour (fifty-four minutes on average) spent waiting.[8] One health care organization estimates that each time a patient (or potential patient) is asked to call a different location from the one originally contacted, 2 percent fail to make the call.

Patients are very aware of these shortcomings and regularly express their displeasure through complaints and satisfaction surveys. As health care becomes more competitive, they are quite willing to switch health plans or providers to obtain better service.

Operational Efficiency and Productivity

Another reason for focusing on access to care is that the traditional local processes for scheduling and registration involve many redundant steps that are ineffective and expensive. Streamlining can bring hefty administrative savings. One hospital calculated that it cost $62.24 for each patient registration. If a patient came in for five procedures, this meant five separate registrations,[9] so streamlining them into a single registration obviously offers substantial reduction in costs.

When loose ends regarding a patient's insurance are not tied up at the beginning of the process, the resulting payment denials involve a great deal of rework, for both the patient and the enterprise. They also result in delays in payment and, sometimes, write-offs. As health care becomes more cost-competitive, these are obvious targets for improvement.

Productivity is another rationale, and a new enterprise scheduling process can improve it in several ways. Last-minute cancellations and patient no-shows for scheduled services waste resources and reduce revenue. Coordinated scheduling that avoids conflicts and supports patients with information and reminders can reduce this lost productivity. Enterprise managers also need access to information on enterprisewide resource availability and utilization, which is inconsistent and difficult to assemble from individual departments. A true enterprise view offers opportunities to improve understanding of demand for services and to manage resources across sites and settings.

Managed Care and Patient Management

Managed care enrollment provides a much more direct way for health care networks to measure patient loyalty than the number of patient visits under fee-for-service health care. The stakes go up as a broader range of services is included in the capitation. Consequently, health care networks with managed care contracts are attuned to trends in reenrollment, and focus groups and satisfaction surveys highlight the importance of access issues to customer loyalty.

In most health care markets, employers monitor patient satisfaction with access; in some they demand better performance as a condition of contract renewal or through associated financial penalties. The Health Plan Employer Data Information Set (HEDIS) measures, developed by the National Committee for Quality Assurance, and other report-card initiatives make it easy for both patients and employers to comparison shop.

Managed care brings other considerations that lead an organization to focus on access. For instance, access to care is the front door to the care system; thus it is the ideal place to initiate population-based management by ensuring that new members are assigned to the appropriate care model, that they receive services appropriate to their health status, and that they are informed about how the care process works. It is also the appropriate leverage point for incorporating demand management initiatives such as primary care triage. The best time to guide new patients to their primary care physician (PCP) or care team for continuity of care is when they initially seek service, and the ideal time to determine whether the request meets the coverage rules of the patient's health plan is when the patient seeks a referral. Dealing with this up front streamlines the process for patients and avoids later surprises (such as claim denials).

Scope and Breadth of New Access Models

A good framework for understanding the new access models is to analyze the scope (what functions the process encompasses) and breadth (what types of settings and services are included) of each type.

Components of Redesigned Process

Organizations working on access to care focus on some or all of the following process components:

Care scheduling: simplifying the scheduling process so that patients can schedule the services they need efficiently and without hassles, managing appointment availability to enterprise standards, and making effective use of scheduled enterprise resources

Integrating patient account management: incorporating reimbursement-related activities into front-end processes to accomplish them in a unified, more timely, and efficient process

Telephone access: providing consistently reliable and timely access for patients who seek care or advice

Creating the ideal patient encounter: organizing and managing the actual patient encounter and the flow through the care system so that patient time obtaining care is minimized and customer service is maximized

Managed care: incorporating health plan–related activities (enrollment and membership) into a unified, more timely, and efficient process

Triage: assisting patients by assessing symptoms and recommending a care strategy that includes self-management or direct care, as appropriate

Medical advice: providing easy access to protocol-based medical advice and health-related information to assist community members in personal health management

Clinical outreach: a range of initiatives geared toward orienting new members, managing demand, and providing proactive outreach

Many of the models incorporate three or more of these components. Organizations that provide at-risk care typically build the largest number of components into their new access process.

As summarized in Exhibit 3.1, all of the process components meet the overriding business drivers of competition in customer service, operational efficiency and productivity, and managed care and patient management in some way. Therefore, organizations that work quite independently are devising similar approaches to their new enterprise processes. Integrating health care systems that compete in similar environments are building new access models that are remarkably similar. Variation arises from different business objectives and from the strategic priority assigned to investing in change rather than from a different vision for the future. In many cases the components not included in an organization's initial model (or the early stages) are on a wish list for future enhancements. This suggests that over time differences will narrow, and an effective access process will be a requirement to remain competitive.

Care Scheduling. Every case example identified in our research involved rethinking care scheduling in some way. As is the case with every new enterprise process, the new perspective comes from thinking about how the enterprise and its customers, rather than individual departments, need the process to work. This inevitably leads to standardization and centralization.

Redesigned processes take a broader view of this component than appointment booking, because making the process work well involves schedule maintenance and preparing both the enterprise and the customer for a successful service encounter. This means that rethinking and change are required beyond just switching to one telephone number.

Patient Account Management. Scheduling and the front end of the patient accounting process are inseparable because their functions are intermingled in practice. From the patient's perspective, scheduling and registration probably appear to be one process.

The rationale for doing a better job with patient registration is quite simple: the most efficient and effective approach is to deal with reimbursement as (if not before) services are scheduled. Once registration is a coordinated enterprise process, it becomes feasible to accomplish registration only once and to include preactivities that formerly occurred at the time of service delivery (for example, co-payment collection).

Telephone Access. Virtually all of the new models redesign telephone access. As health care organizations rethink this component, they are able to import long-standing operating principles from other telephone-based service industries, such as

Pick up calls quickly (and do not lose them).

Have all of the answers necessary to respond to the customer's inquiry. (Never require the customer to call another number.)

Provide "one-stop shopping" (one access point for a broad range of services and information).

Resolve the customer's question or transaction during the first call whenever possible.

Although these principles seem very basic, they were not a management focus in health care until recently.

In creating customer-focused telephone access, health care organizations are also adopting organization and process models that are well established in other service industries.[10, 11, 12, 13] These include call centers that focus exclusively on telephone interactions with customers and that are equipped with telecommunications to manage large volumes of calls. Effective call centers are staffed with well-trained service representatives who can access the information they need, accomplish the necessary business functions on-line, and record the content and outcome of each call. Other lessons that are being adopted by health care include the importance of good listening skills and customer-friendly responses in service representatives. Coaching and incentives that reinforce the quality of customer interactions rather than productivity alone are important as well.

As in other service industries, telephone access is increasingly viewed as a new core business competency for an integrating health care network.[11, 14, 15] This realization leads an increasing number of organizations to create new call centers that facilitate telephone access.

Ideal Patient Encounter. Creating the ideal patient encounter requires taking the customer's view of the experience. Much attention is focused on the waits and delays that patients commonly face, which necessitate some redesign of processes (typically elements of registration). Improving the encounter also requires a new focus on patient flow and tracking, especially in the physician practice environment. Health care organizations often wish to do a better job helping patients find their way around the facility. Encounter redesigns also aim to make patients feel welcome and expected and that the organization has made appropriate arrangements in advance (for example, aides with wheelchairs and interpreters for patients who are not fluent in English).

Some principles are being adopted from other service industries and as a result of research on customers' views on waits and delays. For example, some organizations inform patients when providers are running behind (the principle being that explained waits seem shorter than unexplained waits). When delays exceed

EXHIBIT 3.1. NEW ACCESS MODEL COMPONENTS AND TYPICAL BUSINESS OBJECTIVES THAT INFLUENCE THE DESIGN.

Component	Competition/Customer Service	Operational Efficiency/Productivity	Managed Care/Patient Management
Care Scheduling	• Provide reliable access to care • Meet patient expectations • Improve access for referring physicians • Simplify scheduling of multiple related services	• Improve resource utilization • Achieve labor savings in service centers • Manage resources to meet demand • Reduce cancellations and no-shows	• Meet employer and community standards • Improve member retention • Increase compliance with follow-up care • Guide members to enterprise service providers
Telephone Access	• Meet customer expectations • Ensure reliable and appropriate response • Reduce telephone access points for members	• Facilitate first call resolution • Achieve labor savings in service centers • Improve reporting of customer issues/complaints	• Meet employer and community standards • Improve member retention • Provide one-stop access to services and information for providers • Provide 24-hour, 7 days a week access • Provide access to educational materials for personal health management
Integrate Patient Accounting	• Avoid surprises for patients • Accomplish one-stop update to registration/insurance for patient • Accomplish pre-registration	• Achieve labor savings in service areas and billing/AR • Reduce payment denials • Speed collections • Increase reliability of co-pay collections	• Provide appropriate reimbursement-related activities based on payer type
Ideal Encounter	• Provide one-stop registration • Anticipate and address patient special needs • Reduce waits and delays	• Achieve labor savings in registration • Improve provider productivity • Understand and address bottlenecks • Improve exam room utilization	• Meet employer and community service standards • Improve member retention

Health System **MEMBER** **123-468** Managed Care	• Facilitate access to appropriate care • Simplify referral access • Offer care alternatives to meet patient expectations about access	• Improve PCP panel management • Reduce membership-related calls • Achieve labor savings in claims administration	• Increase appropriateness of utilization • Guide patients to PCP • Simplify referral access • Increase continuity of care • Increase reliability of patient contact information
Triage	• Improve access to information • Avoid unnecessary encounters • Enable personal health management	• Reduce telephone calls to service areas • Reduce unnecessary encounters • Improve communications management for clinicians	• Increase appropriateness of service utilization • Reduce unnecessary emergency and urgent care visits • Improve delivery of one standard of care
Medical Advice	• Serve the community • Provide access to second opinion	• Provide access to enterprise providers • Reduce telephone calls to service areas	• Improve community health status • Improve understanding of community needs
Clinical Outreach	• Achieve patient perception of partnership in wellness management • Reduce need for patients to initiate care	• Achieve labor savings in clinical service areas • Increase productivity of clinicians	• Improve wellness management • Provide reliable and timely follow-up • Substitute telephone care for encounters • Improve patient compliance and personal health management

preset standards, some providers offer care alternatives to their patients (the principle being that customers prefer to play an active role and to perceive that they have some control).[5, 16]

Managed Care Membership. Certain enrollment- and membership-related managed care activities can be made easier for customers and much more efficient for the enterprise if they are integrated into the access process. Like traditional health insurance, managed care has many rules about covered services and authorized providers that are easier to follow as care is being scheduled than to deal with later.

Membership-related activities such as PCP selection, preparation of identification cards, and delivering information on plan benefits can be integrated into the access process. One organization identified seventeen types of member contact points and, for a query involving enrollment or eligibility, nine possible telephone access points in its care system and health plan.[17] Combining these contact points offers efficiency gains for the enterprise and improved customer service for patients. Although networks that operate a health plan can integrate more functions more thoroughly, managed care contracts with outside health plans require local enrollment to engage new patients with their PCPs. Care systems must also manage referrals in accordance with both internal and health plan–defined rules. The incentives to integrate these aspects of managed care grow as the size of the managed care patient population increases.

Triage or Medical Advice. This component is offered by an increasing number of health care organizations, as well as by employers and payers.[14, 15, 18] Basically, it provides patients and community members access to medical advice and information by telephone as an alternative to seeking direct care. Working definitions of triage and medical advice vary considerably and overlap. One way of distinguishing between the two is that triage is symptom-based, whereas medical advice provides general medical information. This distinction does not work in practice, however, because services classified under both names include symptom-based advice and actual patient calls often involve both types of discussion.

In this research, we use the term *triage* when the service is operated in conjunction with, and when patients view it as part of, the care delivery system. We use the term *medical advice* for a broad-based community service offering advice and information. (Some health care organizations provide both a triage service for managed care members and a medical advice service for the community at large.) A practical distinction according to this working definition involves the medical record: triage notes are communicated to the patient's physician or care team and filed in his or her medical record, whereas medical advice notes are not (or are only at the request of the patient).

Triage and medical advice have numerous similarities in practice:

- Clinicians, typically nurses, provide patient advice, although some services also include physicians or clinical pharmacists.

- Interactions with patients who seek advice about how to manage current symptoms are guided by clinical decision support tools.[18, 19, 20]

- Staff can access information about medications or general medical information.

- Conversations with patients are documented, and the documentation is retained for medicolegal reasons.

- Many services offer recorded or printed patient education materials.[14]

- An increasing number of health care organizations offer access to on-line triage, health assessment, and health education resources via the Internet or dial-in access to a Web site.[21, 22, 23]

The remainder of this chapter addresses triage rather than medical advice, because the focus of most IDN activity is on triage.

Clinical Outreach

Clinical outreach represents the intersection between access to care and another new enterprise process—cross-continuum care management, which is discussed in Chapter Six. Taking advantage of the availability of nurses in access centers, clinical outreach includes a variety of patient communication tasks in the routine work of these staff members. This alleviates the confusion and inefficiency of handling patient calls in a busy practice or clinic setting. It also provides proactive outreach to patients that supports them in meeting wellness and disease management goals.

Clinical outreach can include one or more of the following types of patient interactions:

Recording patients who call to leave messages for their PCP (including requests for prescription refills or referrals)

Calling patients either to convey follow-up information (such as laboratory test results) or to assess patient progress

Screening and orienting new members

Providing protocol-based telephone care in place of encounters

Sites and Settings

Business objectives for the process determine how much of the care system—what settings and what services, and in what part of the health network's service area—is folded into the new access process. The coverage ranges from all scheduled services throughout the enterprise to specific services (for example, primary care and triage) within a local service area. Some models fall between these two extremes. Implementation is always staged in some manner, based on region or service areas. Regardless of where an organization begins, its vision for the future usually includes a new access model for all sites and settings.

Emerging Models

As we assembled case examples, it became clear that there is no single ideal model or best practice. Rather, the right fit for each organization results from its business strategy and how that drives the focus on access and the commitment to change, and from its environment (primarily the extent of its organizational integration, how competitive the market has become, and the extent of reimbursement through capitation).

Virtually all of the case examples identified in our research fit one of the three categories shown in Figure 3.2. The new models—common enterprise scheduling, centralized enterprise scheduling, and enterprise access to care—represent three levels of change from the traditional local processes. As indicated, these also represent increasing integration of the process components just discussed. The changes are cumulative, with each model to the right adding new elements. This does not mean that individual organizations evolve through this sequence; rather, most move immediately to a centralized or access-to-care model.

The following description of these new models includes organizational profiles to illustrate how differing environments and business objectives lead organizations to their version of the new enterprise process.

Common Enterprise Scheduling

Common enterprise scheduling creates a single process (with the aid of a common scheduling application) but leaves multiple telephone access points and local governance in place. It involves relatively little organizational change (despite significant challenges in information technology integration and rollout). The net effect—in terms of customer service and operational efficiency—is small in comparison with more aggressive changes. Although there can be other objectives

FIGURE 3.2. SCHEMATIC OF NEW MODELS FOR ACCESS TO CARE.

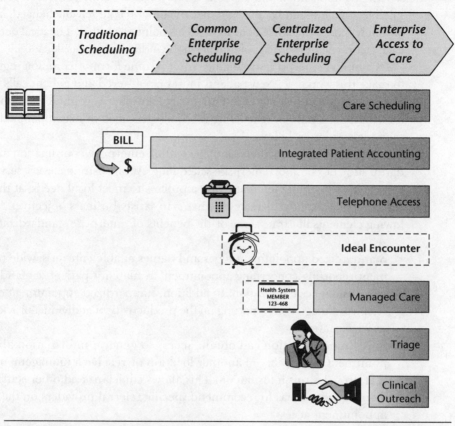

(sometimes information technology objectives) that are important, we did not find this approach being taken in organizations that perceive a strategic need to create new enterprisewide processes for patient care. It comes as no surprise that in the few examples we did find, the organizations were not very integrated.

Process Components. This model involves some aspects of care scheduling and patient account management. Although the procedures for handling patient and other customer calls may be similar, the change is too minimal to count as an improvement in telephone response.

Basic Model. To access care, customers (patients and referring physicians or their staff) call the customary local service areas to schedule appointments and make other arrangements for care, as shown in Figure 3.3. Staff in each location access the same scheduling application and therefore go through the same general steps to find a suitable appointment. For the customer, the process is largely unchanged, although probably more similar from one local access point to another. The ideal outcome of each call is one or more appointments in the individual service location.

Common enterprise scheduling requires some form of common registration to make this workable. New patients must be registered and patient calls must be used to capture updates to basic patient demographic information and insurance information. Common scheduling is usually preceded or accompanied by common registration or billing.

There are two variations on the extent of enterprise coordination and standardization of common enterprise scheduling. At one extreme, every service center sets up scheduling templates and a process to meet local needs; at the other, the enterprise standardizes key elements to satisfy business objectives. The following elements illustrate some of the benefits of enterprise standardization:

- Standardized appointment types and names enable enterprisewide management reporting concerning appointment availability, patient demand for services, and service utilization. In addition, standardized appointment duration enables management reporting on the productivity of individual providers and service locations.
- Staff in one location can obtain access to general information about appointment availability in another location or receive a management report that provides this information. This allows clinicians and other staff in individual service areas to recommend specific referral providers on the basis of appointment access.
- Modern scheduling applications generally support cross-booking of appointments in a different service location, subject to institutional procedures and rules. This means that negotiated cross-booking privileges can be implemented. (These are generally limited, however.)
- Modern scheduling applications also support conflict checking, production of service-specific patient directions and instructions, and mailed and call-out appointment reminders. With sufficient central coordination, these elements can be incorporated into the new process.

Governance. Management remains mostly local, although some enterprise-level coordination is required to fashion a common process. The degree of coordination varies, but extensive coordination is required to achieve standardization of appointment types and names (a prerequisite for many of the business objectives discussed earlier). The focal point for accomplishing this coordination may be a designated manager or committee, typically within the administrative structure.

FIGURE 3.3. COMMON ENTERPRISE SCHEDULING.

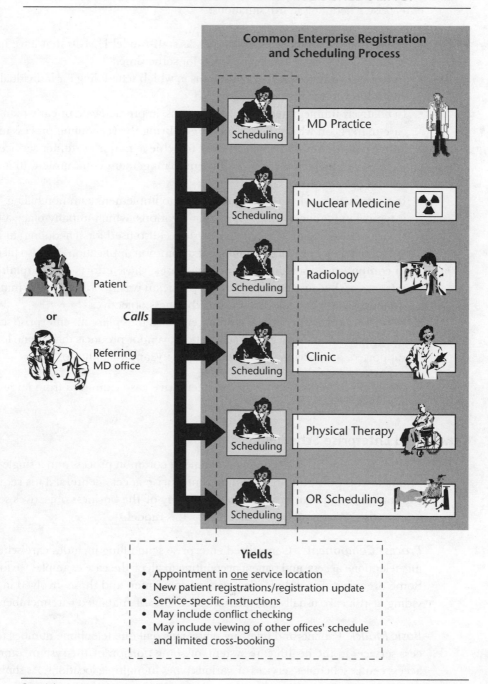

Common Enterprise Registration
and Scheduling Process

Patient

or

Referring
MD office

Calls

Scheduling — MD Practice

Scheduling — Nuclear Medicine

Scheduling — Radiology

Scheduling — Clinic

Scheduling — Physical Therapy

Scheduling — OR Scheduling

Yields

- Appointment in one service location
- New patient registrations/registration update
- Service-specific instructions
- May include conflict checking
- May include viewing of other offices' schedule
  and limited cross-booking

Typical Setting and Business Environment. We found the model for common enterprise scheduling in five situations:

- In integrated care organizations such as staff-model HMOs that have had a common but local scheduling process for some time.[24]
- In relatively unintegrated organizations in which scheduling for individual service areas was largely done manually.[25]
- In relatively unintegrated care organizations, in premanaged or early managed care markets, in which there is a desire to bring the scheduling process under better control but no perceived need to achieve major customer service objectives, or in which there is insufficient management commitment to implement more aggressive change.[26, 27, 28]
- In organizations where the major driver is to implement common billing. This is typical in management services organizations, which initially place a high priority on replacing legacy billing systems (also used for scheduling) in individual physician practices. Rolling out a common application can also fill gaps in computerized scheduling. (In many cases, these efforts do not qualify as *enterprisewide* because they involve only physician practices and require minimal standardization to achieve immediate business objectives.)
- In organizations where there is an urgent need to replace an enterprise scheduling application (homegrown applications, vendor products that are no longer supported, products that cannot handle the year 2000, and so on).

Exhibits 3.2 and 3.3 provide representative case examples from large academic medical centers.

Centralized Enterprise Scheduling

Centralized enterprise scheduling combines a common process and a single telephone access point into one or more enterprise access centers. This requires substantial change but promises to meet many of the business objectives set for new models. We found many examples of this model.

Process Components. Centralized enterprise scheduling includes care scheduling, telephone access, and patient accounting in all of the case examples we found. Some organizations include ideal patient encounter, and those involved in providing at-risk care usually include some elements of managed care membership.

Basic Model. Patients and referring physicians dial one telephone number to access services in the health care system (or some portion of the system), and the access center schedules services of various types in multiple locations. As shown in

EXHIBIT 3.2. COMMON ENTERPRISE SCHEDULING: ALL ENTERPRISE SCHEDULED SERVICES.

Traditional Scheduling → *Common Enterprise Scheduling* → *Centralized Enterprise Scheduling* → *Enterprise Access to Care*

Setting/Environment

- Academic medical center-based health system in an early managed care market.
- The institution had a common registration system and a common, homegrown scheduling system.

Business Objectives

- The overriding objectives were IT-related. The legacy scheduling application was widely recognized as no longer sufficient in terms of its functionality, reliability, and maintainability.
- Rolling out a more function-rich application to all service sites also presented an opportunity to improve local processes and increase overall coordination of scheduling.

Access Model

- Implementation is beginning with physician and procedure-based services on the main campus because of the urgent need to replace the old application. Next will be community-based ambulatory services. Eventually the same process will apply to all scheduled services, including OR and admissions.
- Telephone and other scheduling access points remain local. Staff on inpatient units can call individual service areas to schedule necessary services. Project staff work with a local team to improve the process and ensure that local requirements are met. Enterprise data standards (appointment types and names, etc.) must be adhered to in each service location.
- Patient registrations and registration updates are accomplished during calls. A Verification Unit in Patient Accounting verifies insurance. For managed care patients, service representatives in individual practice and service sites can verify eligibility and coverage during the telephone call with the patient.
- Staff on individual inpatient units call the various practices and service areas to schedule services for inpatients.
- Some service areas were already cross-booking. These are supported in the new common process and new cross-booking agreements are encouraged (but not required).
- Conflict checking, patient instructions and reminders, and scripting for schedulers to ensure that they book the correct service and obtain necessary information will be aggressively implemented with the new application.

Comments

- Increasing integration of the IDN during the course of the multi-year project makes it likely that scheduling will be reorganized and centralized to some extent as a second phase of the project.
- Planned enhancements include direct booking from inpatient units and real-time insurance verification using EDI. Someday, order entry may be linked with scheduling. The organization is considering eventually scheduling inpatient mealtimes so that these can be incorporated into appointment conflict checking.

EXHIBIT 3.3. COMMON ENTERPRISE SCHEDULING: AMBULATORY SERVICES WITH A PHYSICIAN REFERRAL SERVICE.

Traditional Scheduling	Common Enterprise Scheduling	Centralized Enterprise Scheduling	Enterprise Access to Care

Setting/Environment

- Academic medical center with several community hospitals, and employed and affiliated physician practices both on campus and in areas served by community hospitals.
- Common applications and processes are being phased in at physician practice sites, as information technology prerequisites are implemented and the care system increasingly integrates organization and governance.

Business Objectives

- Prior to the rollout, many physician practice sites were still using appointment books. One objective was to improve customer service by providing computerized scheduling in all care sites.
- Difficulty managing the fragmented billing process meant that not all services were billed, and billing errors/payment denials further decreased collections and added administrative cost. Providing a comprehensive encounter database, linked to and reconciled with a new common billing application, was another business objective.
- The enterprise also wanted to offer a centralized physician referral service for physicians.
- Managed care was increasing in the market. A new universal scheduling application would capture encounter information for local and IDN-wide managed care contracts, as well as management information on utilization.

Access Model

- Management and operation of scheduling remain local. The only exception is the physician referral service, which can book new patients into blocked portions of schedules, as negotiated with interested physician practices.
- Implementation included standardization wherever possible to enable management reporting and cross-booking of appointments.
- Working committees representing different disciplines and practices developed standard appointment types and names wherever possible. (Highly specialized services are the least standardized.) Appointment times are still determined within each practice.
- Registration is centralized. Schedulers capture a mini-registration for new patients and offer patients two options: transfer call to Central Registration or complete registration when they appear for care.
- Central Registration is responsible for verifying insurance information.
- Schedulers have access to health plan eligibility and coverage information during scheduling.

Comments

- The design and implementation of a new common registration process. Enterprise redesign projects that focus on customer service and reducing cost are also nearing completion. The next phase of creating an integrated enterprise process will probably lead to pockets of centralization and increased cross-booking (working toward an "ideal" process where community physician offices can directly book initial appointments for referrals).

Figure 3.4, outputs of calls can include one or many coordinated appointments and mailed directions and patient instructions for all scheduled services. When the health care system does not have a suitable appointment available, patients can be referred to alternative care sites or placed on a waiting list. As with common enterprise scheduling, outputs also include patient registrations and updates.

Improving the scheduling process overall is a major objective. This includes redesign and close ongoing management of four elements:

- Patient access to appointments improves with tightly managed schedule maintenance that ensures that the appropriate mix of services and appointment types is available to meet the needs of the population served.
- Efficiency improves as the function is moved out of local service areas to an access center. Service representatives in the center focus exclusively on access-related customer service.
- Customer service is a core element in the new customer-friendly process. In addition to fulfilling the service request, it prepares the patient for the encounter with all necessary directions and instructions, sometimes customized into an agenda for care. Checking for and responding to conflicts at the time of scheduling and establishing policies and procedures for patient reminders limit the occurrence of unnecessary and unproductive visits and missed appointments. The benefit for the enterprise is reduced no-shows and last-minute cancellations.
- A common process with common policies and procedures includes standards for schedule maintenance, as well as appointment types and names across sites and settings. This makes it easier for service representatives to match requests for service with appropriate appointments, and also permits management reporting on an enterprisewide rather than a local basis.

Most of the calls for appointments are routed through a centralized location. The scope of sites and settings covered varies from one center for all hospital-based services in one location to a single access center for all sites and settings in the enterprise.[1, 9, 29, 30] A common middle ground involves regional access centers for large health care networks.[9, 31] In these centers, a closely managed call center focuses on this function, supported by processes and telecommunications familiar in other service industries.

Integration with the front end of patient accounting involves all of the same elements as common enterprise scheduling. In many cases, however, additional patient accounting activities are integrated into the workflow in the access center:

Advising the patient of insurance coverage and personal financial responsibility for the requested services

FIGURE 3.4. CENTRALIZED ENTERPRISE SCHEDULING.

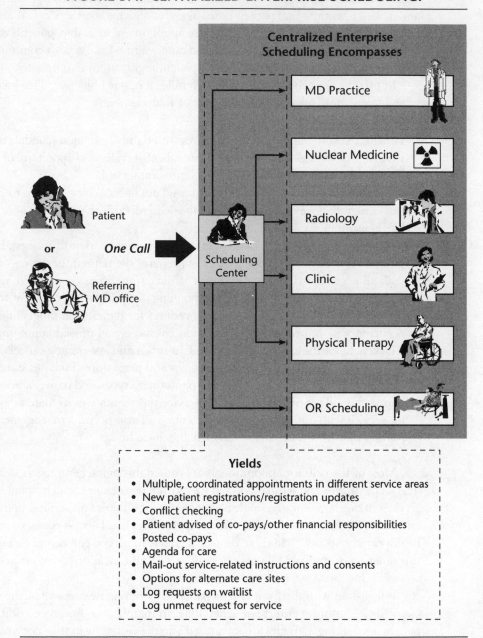

Centralized Enterprise Scheduling Encompasses

Patient

or   *One Call*

Referring MD office

Scheduling Center

MD Practice

Nuclear Medicine

Radiology

Clinic

Physical Therapy

OR Scheduling

Yields

- Multiple, coordinated appointments in different service areas
- New patient registrations/registration updates
- Conflict checking
- Patient advised of co-pays/other financial responsibilities
- Posted co-pays
- Agenda for care
- Mail-out service-related instructions and consents
- Options for alternate care sites
- Log requests on waitlist
- Log unmet request for service

Collecting co-payments, other charges, and unpaid balances over the telephone via credit card

In a few cases, providing financial counseling, as well as information and support for enrolling in public assistance

When the organization is involved in managed care, service representatives typically can look up the patient's PCP and schedule services accordingly. In some cases, service representatives can also assist patients in selecting or changing their designated PCP.

A major goal in integrating patient accounting is to obtain insurance verification and referral authorizations when the service is being scheduled.[9, 32] Difficulties with software application integration or on-line connections with payer databases often require organizations to step back from the ideal process and create work-arounds that they hope to replace over time.

In some organizations, redesign extends to the patient encounter. Typically the changes focus on streamlining registration or check-in and reducing waits and delays.

Governance. Centralized enterprise scheduling is a true enterprise process that cannot be implemented or managed within the traditional management structure. Successful organizations designate an enterprise process owner who typically reports to the chief operating officer (COO) or chief medical officer (CMO), or within a region, to the CEO, COO, or CMO of the region. Specific processes for which the director or manager is accountable typically include both scheduling and registration. Service representatives and other staff who support the access center report to the process owner.

Critical elements of centralized enterprise scheduling are performance standards for elements such as telephone response, appointment access, and patient accounting functions. These are key not only to the basic design but also to staffing and ongoing management. Standards also drive cost and investment. For example, a serious commitment to appointment access may lead to hiring additional staff, extending clinic hours, or opening new call sites to better serve customers. The standards are set and performance is overseen by senior management or a designated steering committee.

Control over the maintenance of schedules is usually centralized; this stems from the importance of meeting enterprise standards and adhering to common policies and procedures.

Settings and Environment. This model is being adopted widely in health care organizations.[1, 9, 29, 30, 31] We found many examples in integrating health networks in competitive markets, and several that defined customer-friendly access as their competitive edge. Exhibits 3.4, 3.5, and 3.6 describe three typical models.

EXHIBIT 3.4. ORGANIZATIONAL PROFILE: CENTRALIZED ENTERPRISE SCHEDULING.

Traditional Scheduling > *Common Enterprise Scheduling* > *Centralized Enterprise Scheduling* > *Enterprise Access to Care*

Setting/Environment
- IDN is in an urban market that has experienced a quick transition to managed care.
- The IDN includes a large number of primary care and specialty practices, as well as a hospital, is relatively integrated, and has a long history of acting as one organization.

Business Objectives
- Customer service has been a long-standing tradition for the organization. The organization relies upon extensive referrals for evaluation, diagnosis, and treatment as a major part of its business. "Customers" include both patients and the office staff of referring physicians.
- Other objectives include pre-registration and pre-verification to the maximum extent possible and guiding managed care patients to the appropriate location for services (PCP or authorized referral specialist, consistent with health plan rules).
- A parallel objective is to have a streamlined, rational, and efficient process so that tasks need be done only once and rework is minimized.

Access Model
- Telephone access from the outside is centralized into one enterprise call center that covers primary care, specialty care and procedures, and any other ancillary services that must be scheduled. A staff of service representatives is supervised by nurses who take calls that require clinical interpretation, but do not triage per se.
- Follow-up appointments and others under specifically-defined circumstances are booked in the individual service areas. Staff in the access center and selected staff in service areas have been trained in the nuances of scheduling and can book "complex appointments." Additional staff in the service areas have had training and are allowed to book simple appointments.
- Service representatives register and record all necessary insurance information for new patients. For managed care patients, they can aid in PCP selection. Verifications and pre-authorizations are handled in a Verification Unit and in Admissions, as appropriate. These are communicated electronically with a goal that they be completed on the same day as the appointment is booked.
- When patients appear for the scheduled care, they check-in once at Central Registration and then proceed to the service area(s).
- Schedule maintenance is the responsibility of staff in the access center. They work with staff in each department to finalize schedules, but build and extend schedule templates centrally.

Comments
- This IDN has developed and implemented numerous business-, clinical-, and physician-specific rules to guide scheduling so that appropriate services are booked and "service representatives never have to guess."
- Eventually, the IDN plans to link order entry with scheduling.

EXHIBIT 3.5. ORGANIZATIONAL PROFILE: CENTRALIZED ENTERPRISE SCHEDULING OF MEDICAL CENTER- AND HOSPITAL-BASED SERVICES.

| *Traditional Scheduling* | *Common Enterprise Scheduling* | *Centralized Enterprise Scheduling* | *Enterprise Access to Care* |

Setting/Environment
- Urban IDN operating in an increasingly competitive, early managed care environment.

Business Objectives
- Customer service was a major objective, in particular the ability to provide one-call access to enterprise services of all types. A corollary objective was to facilitate easy access to appointments for referring physicians.
- Efficiency was another goal, in terms of the efficiencies offered by centralizing a fragmented, local process for both scheduling and insurance verification. A related objective was to incorporate reimbursement-related activity into the front end to avoid rework and payment delays.
- Productivity was also a driver. A more efficient, unified process was expected to match customer service requests with appointments more consistently and improve utilization of enterprise resources across sites and settings.

Access Model
- Telephone access has been centralized into an enterprise scheduling center for hospital-based services.
- Although most scheduling is centralized, the IDN has implemented decentralized access so that staff in each area can view scheduling status at any time, send and receive messages concerning schedules and appointments, and schedule in some cases locally. (The details concerning when and how this is to occur are worked out with each department.)
- The new process was designed to handle insurance verification and authorizations up-front. Sufficient patient information is obtained on the telephone to update or record insurance information, and this is sent in real-time to Patient Accounting. From work lists, staff in Patient Accounting accomplish the necessary verification soon after the appointments are made so that they can contact patients and/or referring physician offices well in advance of the service date to resolve any problems. For patients who call for services such as mammography, a similar procedure (guided by rules about verification depending upon the risk) is followed, and the patient is asked to bring his or her insurance card on the day of service.
- For booking multiple services (e.g., pre-admission testing and assessment), the IDN has created "service sets" and implemented logic in its system to check for conflicts and proper sequencing, include preparation and travel time in assigning appointments, and generate itineraries and maps for patients.

Comments
- The IDN operates a 24-hour nurse advice line, which is not linked to the access center.
- Planned enhancements to the model include an ACD line for physicians and patients to leave messages and an eventual linkage between order entry and scheduling.

EXHIBIT 3.6. ORGANIZATIONAL PROFILE: CENTRALIZED ENTERPRISE ACCESS WITH AREA ACCESS CENTERS FOR HOSPITAL-BASED SERVICES.

| *Traditional Scheduling* | *Common Enterprise Scheduling* | *Centralized Enterprise Scheduling* | *Enterprise Access to Care* |

Setting/Environment

• A multi-hospital in an early managed care market.

Business Objectives

• Provide superior customer service in the market by simplifying and streamlining access.
• Gain efficiencies of centralizing the access process and better success in dealing with requirements for reimbursement by integrating it into the front-end process.
• Prepare for managed care by accomplishing enrollment-driven patient registration and obtaining the necessary authorizations before any services subject to these requirements are delivered.

Access Model

• The model will eventually include all enterprise services. It has begun with hospital-based services because of physician resistance.
• An area Access Center has been implemented for each hospital, and patients call to schedule all hospital-based services. When call response standards are not met, callers are given the option of leaving a message and assured of a prompt call-back.
• When new patients call, service representatives accomplish registration over the telephone. When a physician office refers a new patient, Access Center staff obtain sufficient information for a mini-registration and then call the patient to verify and complete the registration.
• Staff in Patient Accounting verify all insurance information that has not been verified within the preceding 30 days; they also obtain telephone authorizations for services, as required.
• Service representatives are guided by scripts to aid them in matching requests with the correct service and in obtaining any special information needed for the service type. Physician office staff call or fax request information on specially-designed forms that have been distributed to community physicians to clarify the requested service and ensure that other required information is obtained. During off-hours, requests can also be left on voicemail.
• Certain parts of the schedules are reserved for inpatients. Nursing unit staff call the Access Center during the day or put requests into voicemail during off-hours. Service representatives schedule the backlog of requests for inpatient services and other voicemail requests at the beginning of their work day.

Comments

• Planned enhancements include linking scheduling with order entry and direct scheduling of some services by office staff in community physician offices. The IDN also hopes to have service representatives call-out to inactive patients to update registration information.

Not only are health care networks in the process of integrating disparate entities into one enterprise, they are still defining the boundaries of the enterprise through acquisitions and mergers. Given this situation, health care systems tend to start implementing centralized enterprise scheduling in the more integrated portions of the network, in many cases the portion with the most experience operating as an entity. A typical starting point in medical center or hospital-centric organizations is centralized scheduling for hospital-based services. Most often this includes all scheduling of ambulatory diagnostic and therapeutic services and hospital-based physician services. As the examples illustrate, however, the model can include affiliated physician (often specialty) practices that are located on the main campus and perhaps at remote sites as well.

Enterprise Access to Care

Enterprise access to care moves beyond providing access to the services characteristic of centralized enterprise scheduling to add new clinical elements and create a new front end to the care system. This model is the most cross-functional and involves the most change from traditional processes. It is found today in organizations that have had the most experience with at-risk care, especially those that operate their own health plans.

Many of the other organizations identified in our research are redesigning care management to eventually incorporate the same types of clinical outreach. Thus we are confident that this component of enterprise access to care represents the future for integrated delivery systems. The potential appears to be enormous, and we are clearly in the early stages of understanding how to fully leverage the access process in the interest of proactive management of large populations of patients.

Process Components. The enterprise access process includes all of the components of centralized enterprise scheduling. In addition, care management functions are integrated into the routine workflow of the access center, and with these functions clinicians—typically nurses—work alongside access service representatives. Some organizations include managed care membership-related functions in addition to those found in centralized enterprise scheduling.

Basic Model. Enterprise access to care provides one-call access to a spectrum of services and information (see Figure 3.5). Typically one access center serves the enterprise or several centers handle large service areas. In addition to service representatives, triage nurses are on hand to manage calls with clinical content. Usually telephone access to triage is provided twenty-four hours a day, seven days a week.

FIGURE 3.5. ENTERPRISE ACCESS TO CARE.

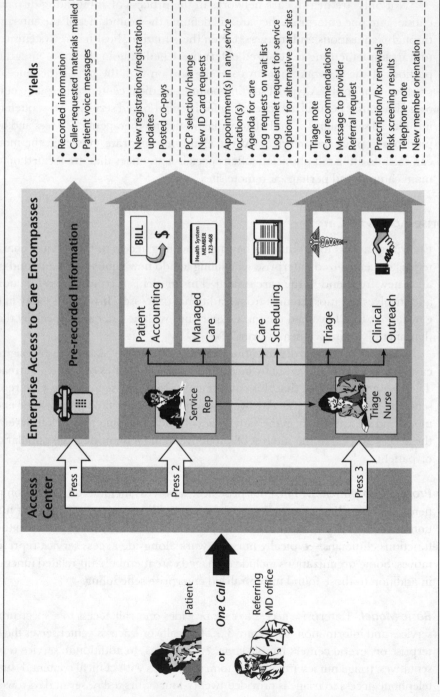

Triage is the most likely patient management function to be integrated into the access process, always paired with appointment scheduling for primary care. Some health care systems offer triage as a separately managed (and located) service,[31] but such arrangements generally pre-date an enterprise access process. Integrating triage offers several advantages:

- Service representatives can refer callers to a triage nurse, which eliminates the need for placing a separate telephone call. (This can be useful for targeting certain types of patient and care situations.)
- Triage nurses can book necessary appointments for primary care and other services. This can take the place of a separate process for referral management when the indications for acute or specialty care are obvious.
- Communication between triage nurses and PCPs, primary care case managers, and clinical teams is enabled by electronic mail and shared enterprise applications such as an ambulatory patient care system. This provides better information for triage and permits triage notes to be documented directly into the patient's electronic health record.
- Triage nurses are available to perform additional care management initiatives.

Triage is enabled by decision support tools that guide the nurse through the patient conversation and documentation of the call. Numerous protocols are required to accommodate the many types of complaints that callers can report. These are indexed to symptom (for example, sore throat or rash) or diagnosis (for example, influenza) and separately developed for different age groups (for example, pediatric or geriatric).

Two different styles of tools are employed. Protocols list general considerations for the nurse that aid in determining the appropriateness and urgency of care. Algorithms provide more customized triage by guiding the nurse through a detailed review of the caller's circumstance, including branching logic based on information provided by the patient, and leading to more specific recommendations for self-care or level and source of care.[14, 20] (Chapter Five contains an example of algorithm-based triage.) Nurses who employ either type of decision support tool would benefit from the opportunity to review patient information such as medications, problem list, and encounter history. We found very few cases in which information technology had advanced to this point, but this is clearly the ideal.

The triage note should be immediately available to the PCP or patient care team and be incorporated into the patient's medical record.[19] Immediate availability is especially useful when the outcome of triage is an appointment for service or a callback from the patient's PCP. (To support continuity of care in this way is another rationale for integrating triage into the access model.) Organizations that do not yet have electronic linkage or automated medical records typically fax triage notes to physicians. (In triage services that operate separately from the health care system, notes are often communicated to physicians only with patient authorization.[20])

In some access centers, triage nurses handle a variety of patient requests and communication. Most common are messages to the PCP for prescription renewals or call-backs. (Urgent calls are connected immediately with the practice site or clinic.) We also learned of one access center where triage nurses, who could review patients' electronic records on-line, could approve prescription renewals for patients who met specified criteria (for example, a renewal of a medication for control of hypertension if the patient had a visit that included a blood pressure check within a specified time frame) and prescribe medications under certain circumstances (for example, if called-out microbiology results confirm streptococcal infection). Referral requests from patients can also be recorded (including all pertinent information) for transmission to the physician.

True outreach is achieved when triage nurses make outgoing telephone calls to members. We identified quite a range of types of call-outs—for example, to notify patients who have had a recent encounter (hospital discharge or ambulatory surgery care) of specified types of laboratory results,[2, 14, 15] to check on the status of patients who have had a recent triage interaction (referred to emergency care), to check on patient status at the request of a clinician, to welcome and orient new members, to screen new members for immediate health needs and possible enrollment in a chronic disease management program,[18, 33] to check periodically with members enrolled in such programs to assess status and compliance and coach in self-management, and to contact inactive members who have had no documented interaction with the care system for some period of time. We found a number of organizations that had far greater ambitions for clinical outreach than could be implemented with current information technology.

In addition to triage, some organizations have reported substituting a different type of service for a traditional encounter. One approach uses prearranged telephone follow-up by a nurse in place of a recheck office visit. In one example in which follow-up of patients with minor trauma was accomplished by telephone, recheck visits were reduced and more than 90 percent of patients were satisfied with the level of service.[34] Another innovation involved prearranged telephone contact with elderly patients with chronic diseases in place of more frequently scheduled clinic visits; the researchers concluded that telephone care reduced utilization without adversely affecting patient health.[35]

Another approach uses protocols for telephone management in place of an office visit to assess patient problems and initiate treatment. A good example of this is the treatment protocol for simple cystitis in adult women that was developed by the Institute for Clinical Systems Integration and implemented in some of its member organizations.[36] For patients who meet specific selection criteria, a nurse prescribes a course of antibiotics rather than requiring a physician visit and routine urine culture to confirm the diagnosis. This has reduced utilization of urine cultures without decreasing clinical outcomes. (Chapter Five includes an illustration of how a triage nurse would administer this protocol.)

As organizations gain more experience with these types of clinical initiatives and as information technology support makes it feasible to implement them for large numbers of patients, we expect that many such protocols will be incorporated into routine practice in enterprise access centers.

Governance. Enterprise access to care is a highly cross-functional process that extends even into the realm of care management. In addition to requiring an enterprise process owner, this model requires either a matrix or line relationship with the patient management process. Models identified so far tend to count access as patient care rather than administrative process and place it under the enterprise medical director. We found two large health care systems with access medical directors, in recognition of the significance of the clinical content being integrated into the access process, as well as the need for extensive ongoing coordination with care delivery and clinical practice initiatives.

Settings and Environment. Our research uncovered numerous examples of integrated triage but only a few examples of clinical outreach. Many organizations, however, are headed in this direction. The major distinction between those that are evolving to this model and those that are actually operating it today is whether or not they can incorporate physician services—primary care in particular—into the new enterprise process. Clear prerequisites are close business affiliation with (if not ownership of) physician practices and the shared business interest of at-risk care. Another prerequisite is time to assimilate acquired practices and build the structure and organization within which an enterprisewide patient care process can be designed and implemented. Exhibit 3.7 describes a typical access model focused on triage and primary care.

Organizational Challenges

Access to care is almost always the first serious attempt to design and implement an enterprisewide process. The difficulties encountered are harbingers of the organizational challenges that will accompany any new patient care process that spans traditional departments and sites of care.

EXHIBIT 3.7. ENTERPRISE ACCESS TO CARE: AREA ACCESS CENTERS FOR AMBULATORY CARE AND TRIAGE.

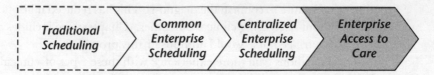

Setting/Environment

- Delivery system with an HMO in an advanced managed care market.
- Access considerations have become a requirement for member re-enrollment and employer contracting, rather than merely a competitive advantage.

Business Objectives

- Use the highly customer-focused access process as a strategic advantage. A corollary objective is to provide "world-class" customer service.
- Achieve local operating efficiencies in service areas by streamlining and coordinating member telephone access to services and information.
- Improve demand management by incorporating triage and other clinical initiatives into the front-end process.
- Increase continuity of care by communicating triage interactions to direct care teams in primary care and urgent care sites.
- Increase member access to specialty services by incorporating referral guidelines and authorization into the front-end process.

Access Model

- Area access centers throughout the service area provide members with one-call access to services and information. Access centers are staffed with service representatives, triage nurses, physicians, and pharmacists to handle the range of member requests. Area centers are linked so that call overflow can be routed to another center as necessary to meet telephone response standards. Urgent or emergency calls can be transferred to the patient's care team.
- Callers are given the choice of speaking with a service representative or triage nurse, or gaining access to pre-recorded information on a broad range of health topics. For targeted clinical situations, service representatives transfer calls to triage nurses. Triage nurses can route calls to physicians or pharmacists, as appropriate to the subject matter of the caller's question or health issue.
- Appointments can be booked for primary care, urgent care, and specialty care sites. Member-requested consults are managed according to protocols that permit self-referral and pre-authorized referrals in designated situations. Triage nurses can pre-authorize emergency and acute care when warranted.
- Triage nurses perform protocol-based call-out and new member orientation, as well as handling incoming calls.
- All patient interactions with the access center are documented and available to clinicians in service sites. Members can leave messages requesting prescription renewals or a call-back from their PCP or care team. They can also select or change their designated PCP.

Comments

- Access centers operate seven days a week, around the clock.
- Clinical initiatives that have been incorporated into the access centers are enabled by electronic access to patient information both in the access centers and care sites and by electronic messaging.

Centralization

Business objectives relating to customer service and efficiency drive models to centralization of patient access points and functions. Virtually all of the new models identified in this research include substantial centralization, although this does not always mean centralization for the entire enterprise. Variations include centralization within a service region or area of the health care system, as well as centralization within a large care site. Modern telecommunications technology enables "virtual centralization," whereby one access center can handle overflow calls or manage the entire call volume in the event of a major system failure or emergency.

Many new models centralize registration to enhance customer service or as part of a parallel enterprise initiative to create a common or a minimal number of common billing processes. Scheduling and registration/billing are therefore entwined in the process and in data management, so some changes to these processes are inevitable, regardless of the business objectives that drive the change.

Resistance to Centralization. Resistance to centralization is probably the greatest institutional challenge in implementing models of new access to care. One project manager who has had several years of experience in opening regional patient access centers describes the feeling of "always walking up a steep mountain with a heavy backpack while everyone else in the organization is moving boulders into the path." This is particularly difficult when (as is often the case) the organization is in transition and still building the structure and culture of one enterprise.

Resistance is understandable because patient contact and scheduling are the major intake processes for a business and are therefore "core" processes. The degree of control lost by local managers and staff is further compounded if the new access model incorporates patient account management (for example, entry and updates to insurance information, insurance verification, and collection of co-payments), because these affect billing and collections.

Concerns about centralization usually include both genuine disbelief that it can work ("No one can provide the same level of service to my patients," or "We have many unique requirements that a centralized process could never accommodate") and discomfort with the loss of control. Physicians are predictably resistant, as are managers of departments that require coordination of multiple resources to schedule services (for example, radiology services and the operating room). Every organization we identified in our research that is planning or implementing centralized enterprise scheduling or enterprise access to care reports major resistance.

Centralization may be somewhat easier to accomplish in health care systems that are more structurally integrated, but staff in organizations that appear to be relatively integrated (at least to outsiders) also report great resistance. Resistance is a universal reality that must be addressed.

Overcoming Resistance. A clear grounding in the enterprise business strategy and a consensus about business objectives are prerequisites for aggressive reorganization of the access process. This leads to a management push to overcome resistance and the sustained investment of resources required to design, implement, and manage a new access process that works.

For many participants, a pilot and initial roll-out are needed to demonstrate not only that the new process can function but also that it provides value to all stakeholders. Many organizations set expectations for improvements and use these to gauge progress and demonstrate value to skeptics. This sets a high bar for success, but a realistic one, because the front-end process is mission-critical and the whole organization can be shut down if it fails to work properly.

Several enterprise access project managers pointed out that physicians in particular adopt a show-me attitude but are won over by demonstrated value to their patients and efficiency in the practice or clinic. Often, however, they have an excessively optimistic view of how well the baseline processes work. Organizations rarely (if ever) have good information on performance, especially concerning telephone response and access to appointments. In several cases where baseline performance was documented in special studies during redesign, physicians and other participants, shocked by the current level of service, became much more predisposed toward radical change.

Physicians and their business managers understand the hassles, delays, and administrative overhead of reimbursement, with both fee-for-service and managed care. They generally welcome improvements that shift this burden and reduce aggravation for themselves, as well as for patients. Including these improvements in the front-end process to minimize surprises and rework can help to overcome the natural resistance to surrendering local control.

Another strategy that we observed in several cases was an effort to incorporate into the redesigned process specific features that minimize the appearance of change. Different telephone numbers and preferential call routing can be used to connect callers who seek services in a particular service location (for example, a specific primary care practice or physician) to a small subset of the service representatives and triage nurses in the access centers.[19, 32] With computer-telephony integration, access center staff can even receive prompts on their computer workstations alerting them to answer the phone by saying "Dr. _____'s office, may I help you?" This permits patients to interact with familiar access center staff and for the staff to become familiar with frequent callers. Several health care systems further reinforced the feeling of continuity (both for patients and for service area staff) when they encouraged displaced scheduling and reception staff to apply for job openings in the access center.

Centralization and Decentralization

Most of the identified models retain some decentralized functions, as well as centralization of the access point for most incoming telephone calls. This typically includes the ability to view service schedules and often the ability to book urgent or follow-up encounters. Customer service goals in particular are not served if, at the conclusion of encounters, rather than being assisted at the care site so that they leave with appointments in hand, patients are told to call a particular central number. We identified one case in which the major dissatisfaction with area access centers for primary care and triage was the inability to book follow-up appointments at practice sites. Unfortunately the scheduling application used was unable to accommodate decentralized scheduling. An added inducement to permit decentralized scheduling is that patient compliance with recommended follow-up care may increase.[37]

A process that includes centralized and decentralized activities is obviously a great deal more complicated to manage. The most complex design we encountered with respect to the boundaries between centralization and decentralization is described in the organizational profile in Exhibit 3.4.

Schedule Maintenance

With centralized scheduling, IDNs often centralize schedule maintenance.[30, 38] The rationale is to ensure that schedules are built and maintained in accordance with enterprise standards. In addition to creating standards for appointment types and times, centralized schedule maintenance addresses issues such as hours of service and the scheduling horizon (that is, how far in the future schedules are open for booking). It turns out that all of this becomes more coordinated and consistent when the function of schedule maintenance is centralized. At Lahey Clinic in Burlington, Massachusetts, for example, five full-time scheduling coordinators maintain schedules for more than four hundred clinicians and twenty-eight departments.[30] This does not mean that clinical service lines and ancillary department managers are not involved—scheduling coordinators work closely with staff and management in their assigned service areas on a daily basis, and service line chiefs sign off on schedules before they are extended.[30]

Standardization

A common process that substitutes for diverse local processes is an essential element of all new models for access to care. This is a prerequisite for realizing many of the core business objectives for the new process, which include the following:

- A truly customer-friendly process should be consistent for patients regardless of where in the health care system they seek access and what types of services or assistance they require.

- Part of the solution to appointment availability is simplifying and standardizing appointment types, which provides greater flexibility to match requests with open appointments.

- Process standardization across care settings (and in some cases, regions) is required before operations can be managed to corporate performance standards, and before performance measurements are meaningful.

Scheduling processes in particular are very complex, and one of the challenges in redesign is to achieve a balance between desirable local variation and essential standardization (that is, to determine what must be standardized to meet business objectives). Because most new models take control of the core access process away from staff in individual care sites, retaining local flexibility to the maximum extent consistent with corporate objectives is a critical success factor.

Standardization of the process from the patient's perspective, for key data elements such as service names and appointment types and otherwise as necessary to meet corporate objectives, was common to all the identified models of centralized enterprise scheduling and enterprise access to care. This appears to be a reasonable working definition of the bare minimum of what needs to be standardized. Several of the organizations we identified stopped short of standardizing appointment times.

Standardizing service names and appointment types and names is not a trivial task. Many project managers reported that some of the most heated debate revolved around true versus perceived differences and the trade-offs between simplification and specificity. Physician and radiology services appear to be particularly problematic. During its redesign of access to primary care and triage, one organization managed to create five or six standard appointment types from a starting point of two hundred![19] Another site determined that physician services could be accommodated by two types of appointments: long and short (with appointment duration times defined differently for primary care and individual specialty disciplines).[5]

Enterprise policies and procedures must be defined to replace the myriad of local policies, procedures, and practices that have evolved in every health care organization. Once again, these should relate to those aspects of the process that are standardized, but they should also mesh with processes and procedures that remain under local control.

Important standardizing elements for the triage and medical advice components of new access models are the algorithms or protocols that guide the advice nurse and other staff who provide information and instructions to patients. Similarly, clinical initiatives aimed at demand management and clinical outreach are guided by protocols and decision support tools to ensure uniform application and reinforce a single standard of care.

Change Management

All new models that centralize the access process involve substantial change. The more components that are included, the greater will be the change, because of ripple effects that occur elsewhere in the care system. Major rethinking and re-design are required to encompass both the new centralized access process and all of the many service areas from which the activities have been centralized and integrated. This means that virtually all front-end processes (in-bound telephone calls, registration, managed care enrollment, scheduling, check-in), as well as many aspects of patient management and follow-up, billing, and claims administration, can be transformed or affected in some way.

Organizations with successful projects work hard to ensure that the needs and expectations of all stakeholders are met in the redesign. Many of the organizations that involved patients in the process through focus groups report that there is a danger in relying on institutional interpreters for patient interests (especially physicians), because surprises often emerge when they investigate how patients actually view the many trade-offs. We also found that organizations all look for successful models, both within and outside of health care, for good practices to emulate as well as for proof of feasibility in the health care setting.

Several project managers emphasized the need for a comprehensive understanding of the procedures and issues associated with each type of service area so that all of the necessary details are addressed in the redesign.[1] One manager from a health care system that is building a centralized scheduling process for the entire enterprise described spending a full year observing and discussing operations in radiology departments, the surgical suite, and physician practices before finalizing plans for an enterprise access process. She stressed the need to "obsess about the details" to get it right.

New access models also bring major changes for patients who have long been accustomed to the decentralized legacy processes. Several project managers stressed the need to involve everyone in the enterprise in explaining to patients and reminding them of the new procedures. Personal communication should be supplemented by newsletters, internal posters, and other methods of disseminating the information. They also reported the importance of visiting referring physician practices to explain the new procedures, distribute new forms and instruction sheets, and discuss other implications of the change.

Implications for Staffing

Job descriptions for service representatives and triage nurses are extremely broad, given the integration of many traditionally separate processes into the new enterprise access process. In addition, the new jobs come with explicit requirements for providing a high level of customer service. Organizations typically must write totally new job descriptions that emphasize these customer service skills, as well as the cross-functional nature of the jobs. When staff from local service areas are redeployed, not all are able to handle the variety and complexity of the work, especially the interactive use of computers to handle so many different tasks.

Detailed policies and procedures, extensive training (sometimes for as much as twelve to sixteen weeks), and supervision are required. We identified numerous cases where many customer interactions were scripted for front-line staff, used in training, and displayed on computer terminal screens to guide actual patient interactions. As in other service industries, employee performance should be judged on quality as well as productivity (the number of calls taken or made). To this end, coaching and recording samples of actual calls for review and discussion are becoming common practices. Close supervision in the access center can require one supervisor for every five or six service representatives.

Operating high-technology call centers represents a whole new skill area for health care. The lack of in-house expertise is one reason that some organizations outsource triage or medical advice services to a national service organization.[20] Those that operate their own access centers often recruit call center management and operations staff from other service industries.

Process Governance and Management

Access to care is typically the first new enterprisewide process to be instituted. Therefore, to implement a new model an organization must confront a dizzying array of challenges that are associated with creating integrated enterprise processes: Who is the process owner? Where does the process owner fit in the organization chart? Where does the budget fit? How will the process be managed and governed? How will management of the access process be coordinated with other enterprise processes? It is no surprise that rolled-out enterprise processes are found only in organizations that have addressed these questions (at least to some extent).

Process Ownership. For true enterprise processes, we found owners for enterprise scheduling, scheduling and registration, or access to care (or the equivalent by a different name) who report to the enterprise executive team (through the COO or CMO for the enterprise). In organizations with regionally focused management structures, each region has an owner for the access process (regardless of how it is defined).

Creating and implementing the new enterprise structure and organization takes time—sometimes years, as discussed in Chapter One. We found one organization in which the new owner of enterprise scheduling and registration was actually rolling out a new centralized enterprise model for hospital-based services before new management structures were in place at the individual sites. Each new access center had a manager who reported up through the old management structure, as did the service representatives. The process owner described her job as entailing a combination of pushing, persuading, and anything else that worked to keep things moving forward and meeting enterprise objectives. (She indicated that a good sense of humor helped, too.) We know that this transitional hybrid of local and enterprise processes is not unique.

Models we have classified as enterprise access incorporate care management functions. In all identified examples, clinicians (with physician leadership and interdisciplinary representation) designated by the IDN's medical director were in charge of managing clinical content. In fact, the ability to organize and empower such a group is prerequisite to incorporating patient management into the access process. This role includes the selection, review, and customization of software applications such as triage software and patient educational materials that may be purchased from vendors, as well as in-house-developed protocols and guidelines. As with other clinical practice initiatives, this role includes periodic updating to reflect changes in clinical practice.

Matrix Management. Even with a designated enterprise-level process owner, matrix management is required for new models of enterprise access. In the case of centralized enterprise scheduling, this management results from the combination of centralized and decentralized access-related activity and the integration of at least some portion of the front end of patient accounting into the process. The inclusion of patient management functions and managed care membership in models for enterprise access to care adds at least two more enterprise processes to the mix.

The organization profiled in Exhibit 3.4 provides an interesting example of how the management structure can evolve as the organization gains experience. Initially, decentralized schedulers and other cross-trained staff reported to the enterprise process owner because their function was viewed as part of the enterprise process. Supervising so many distributed personnel presented a real challenge for the process owner. Over time the organization's senior management decided that teamwork within a department or physician's practice would be enhanced if the decentralized staff were managed locally, and they revised the structure accordingly.

To coordinate with local operations, the process owner instituted regular meetings with local physicians, practice managers, and local scheduling staff. According to the process owner, there were significant trade-offs with either approach.

Management to Standards. With a focus on customer service, new models of access to care are managed to meet enterprise performance standards. In fact, some organizations start the redesign effort by developing performance expectations for the new process (including specific levels) and then design the organizational and process model required to deliver that level of customer service. We found the most consistent focus to be on standards relating to appointment access and telephone response, but we also found an increasing interest in process and outcome metrics for other components of new models.

Many organizations employ patient focus groups to incorporate the patient's perspective in enterprise performance standards. Some competitor information may be available for a few measures of performance, but generally health care organizations determine the standards of service they wish to deliver and define specific metrics to be meaningful for internal use. Over time, the influence of HEDIS and other report card initiatives will increase the standardization of both performance metrics and data definitions for constructing the metrics. Until that standardization occurs, it will be difficult (and even misleading) to compare performance across organizations.

Few organizations managed access processes in this way in the past (or if they attempted to do so they were unable to obtain consistent and reliable performance reporting). Developing, approving, and managing to enterprise standards is a new activity. Standards are set and sanctioned at the enterprise level, typically by (or with sign-off from) the executive team. Ongoing management to meet standards is obviously key. The HMO Group study of best practices confirmed that higher-performing sites not only had a process for performance measurement but also reviewed and acted on performance information frequently.[3]

Migration to New Models

For multi-institution, integrated processes, full rollout can take as long as three to five years. Given the scope of organizational change and the need to coordinate with other enterprise initiatives, implementation is typically conducted in phases. For each institution, local business drivers and environmental factors determine where implementation starts and how it proceeds.

Every organization starts with a pilot (although use of the term *pilot* is often discouraged because it implies that the initiative is optional or the organization is not yet committed to the change). Pilots provide an opportunity to reality-test the new process and enabling information technology. They can also function as a "proof of concept" that builds consensus within the organization that the new model works and provides the intended value. In any case, the choice of location and process scope for the pilot is critical. The effort must be substantial enough to provide a good test, but also reasonable and feasible. (A positive outcome is critical to moving forward.)

Pilots and subsequent rollout phases become the new process for the affected service locations and patients because it is not possible to run parallel old and new processes. One fundamental principle in designing pilots and subsequent rollout is that the new process must always make sense to, and provide value for, the affected patients and physicians—it must not further fragment or complicate the process. As a result, pilots include most if not all of the elements in the model. When rollout is staged, this means that substantial elements of the new model must be rolled out together.

The combination of environmental factors, business drivers, and the baseline information infrastructure can lead to very different rationales on where to begin. During benchmarking we encountered all of the following strategies:

- Start where we can make the biggest difference for patients and for the enterprise (often primary care).

- First fix areas with demonstrated poor performance (also often primary care or specific primary care practices).

- Initially focus on locations that provide convincing proof of concept.

- Start where it is possible to accomplish all key portions of the new model.

- Focus on areas that currently lack information technology, because they are most in need of help and the easiest to implement.

- Start with services or physician practices that have the poorest performance records.

- Start with the most integrated portion of the care system, such as staff physicians, practices, or hospitals that have new enterprise management structures to govern and manage the new enterprise process.

- Start with rollout of the standard application and standard practices, but maintain local processes to give the organization time to learn and adjust; then proceed with centralization.

- Drive the rollout from plans for related corporate initiatives such as common registration or a master patient index.

The last point is always critical because access to care is typically the first enterprise process, and initiatives such as registration or a master patient index are usually gating factors for rollout.

Migration plans reflect very different approaches to the pacing and scope of change, as illustrated by the following examples.

• *IDN that operates a health plan.* Redesign and implement primary care and triage in regional call centers. Use pilot for proof of concept and to learn about the scheduling application and the challenges of implementation and operation, then roll out to additional regional centers. Move in parallel on centralized scheduling for hospital-based services (mostly on-campus in medical centers). When established, consider linkage and use of a specialty service center to handle call overflow from primary care scheduling center.

• *Multisite group model HMO implementing a common patient care system.* Roll out standardized enterprise registration and scheduling, with enterprise standards for appointment types, names, and so on, but leave decentralized triage and scheduling in place initially. Start cross-practice and site booking where there is a clear business rationale—for example, weekend triage nurses booking urgent appointments for the following Monday, or family practice booking initial obstetrical appointments for pregnant patients who elect to have their care in obstetrics. When a national HMO arrived in the market, this HMO faced the need to cut costs substantially or increase productivity; the medical staff preferred to centralize scheduling (and thereby realize administrative staff savings) over other measures proposed, such as increasing physician schedule hours. Centralized scheduling was a big success with physicians, other providers, and patients; the next step was centralizing triage to the same location.

• *Urban IDN including several hospitals and outlying physician practices.* Management was committed to centralizing registration and scheduling in a customer-friendly process. The steering committee for the redesign and implementation decided that the most effective way to demonstrate feasibility and value to the institution was to tackle the most complicated services to schedule (operating room, radiology, and rehabilitation services such as physical and occupational therapy) and the physician group most difficult to please (surgeons). After a successful rollout in the medical center, they added the same services in several community hospitals in order to benefit from cross-site booking to meet patient demand for services (which was most useful for radiology). Further plans include the remaining hospital-based services in the enterprise process and, finally, outlying physician practices.

• *Regional HMO.* Focus on primary care and triage because of their importance to patient satisfaction, demand management, and area employers. Pilot with one regional call center as a learning experience and then roll out others. Defer redesign and implementation of the new process for specialists and hospital-based services.

Conclusions and Predictions

There is no single model or best practice for enterprise access. However, when the emerging models are categorized into the typical patterns identified in our research, there is surprisingly little scatter in the business objectives set by integrating health networks and the models they design to meet those objectives. We believe that this can be explained by the consistent business drivers and environment accompanying at-risk care and the adoption of principles and practices of good customer service from other industries. This means that our picture of the future process in integrated care delivery is quite clear.

The focus on customer service in health care is here to stay. Competition—in cost and performance—is a new fact of life. As we have seen in other service industries, customer service, during both telephone interactions and encounters, becomes a major basis for differentiation among competitors. Now that health care is competitive and so many organizations are offering (or will soon offer) better access, the focus on customer service will become universal in any market with significant penetration of managed care.

Customer service is tangible for patients and an area they feel competent to judge. The report card movement is providing ready access to comparative information on which health care customers will rely increasingly as input for decisions about where to seek services. Over time, the combination of increasing customer orientation in health care and the rising standards for customer service in other industries will raise the bar for customer service in health care.

Implementing new enterprise models is expensive and painful because it involves enormous change and a shift away from traditionally local control over critical and sensitive processes. The transformation is difficult and the resistance is strong, even in organizations that are relatively integrated and that share a sense of common business purpose. We do not believe that loosely affiliated networks will have the management commitment or staying power to create centralized and integrated models that provide the requisite level of customer service. Loosely affiliated health care networks will have difficulty competing on the basis of access management.

Access to care is the front end of patient management. Integration into the access process is a requirement for managing care. Many organizations are implementing centralized enterprise scheduling in early managed care markets. As these organizations gain more experience with providing at-risk care, we believe they will enhance their access process to incorporate at least some of the elements we see today in the model for enterprise access to care.

Notes

1. Morrissey, J. "The Perfect Fit: Computerized Patient Scheduling Requires the Right Mix of Software, Hardware, and Human Components." *Modern Healthcare,* 1996, *26,* 56–62.

2. Morrissey, J. "On Call: Foundation Health Systems' Sophisticated Telephone Triage Center Gains Popularity with Patients and Physicians." *Modern Healthcare,* 1997, *27,* 72–76.

3. Joshi, M. S. "Improving the Appointment Scheduling Process: A National, Multi-HMO Benchmarking Initiative." *HMO Practice,* 1994, *8,* 180–184.

4. Nolan, T., and Schall, M. W. *Guide to Reducing Delays and Waiting Times Throughout the Healthcare System.* Boston: Institute for Healthcare Improvement, 1996.

5. Institute for Healthcare Improvement. *National Congress on Reducing Delays and Waiting Times in Health Care.* Boston: Institute for Healthcare Improvement, 1996.

6. *1997 Environmental Assessment: Redesigning Health Care for the Millennium.* Irving, Texas: VHA, Deloitte & Touche, 1997.

7. Sachs, M. A., and Pickens, G. T. "What Members Want." *HMO Magazine,* 1997, *36,* 21–24.

8. Borowitz, S. M. "Impact of a Computerized Patient Tracking System in a Pediatric Clinic." In J. J. Cimino (ed.), *1996 AMIA Fall Annual Meeting.* Philadelphia: Hanley & Belfus, 1996.

9. Cross, M. A. "Patient Scheduling Made Easy." *Health Data Management,* Aug. 1996, pp. 65–67.

10. *An Exchange of Knowledge Among Leading Practitioners in Customer Management.* Cambridge, Mass.: Arthur D. Little, 1994.

11. Rappaport, D. M. "The Press for More Options." *CIO,* 1997, *10* (1), 30–34.

12. Cooperstein, D. "Click Here for an Agent." *CIO,* 1997, *10* (1), 36–37.

13. Nash, J. "Fast Fone Farms, Fat Profits." *CIO,* 1997, pp. 40–52.

14. Prescott, M. "A Friendly Voice in the Night." *Healthplan,* 1996, *37,* 47–53.

15. Appleby, C. "Speed Dialing." *Hospitals and Health Networks,* 1997, *71,* 58–60.

16. Czepiel, J. A., Solomon, M. R., and Surprenant, C. F. *The Service Encounter: Managing Employee/Customer Interaction in Service Businesses.* Lexington, Mass.: Heath, 1985.

17. Pietrick, A. G. "Health Maintenance Organization: Reengineering Member Services." In P. Boland (ed.), *Redesigning Healthcare Delivery: A Practical Guide to Reengineering, Restructuring, and Renewal.* Berkeley, Calif.: Boland Healthcare, 1996.

18. Lester, J. A., and Breudigam, M. "Nurse Triage Telephone Centers: Key to Demand Management Strategy." *NAHAM Management Journal,* Spring 1996, pp. 13–34.

19. Anctil, B., and Winters, M. "Linking Customer Judgments with Process Measures to Improve Access to Ambulatory Care." *Journal of Quality Improvement,* 1996, *22,* 345–357.

20. Nobel, J. J., and Gill, M. "Cost Reduction Through Telecomputing-Supported Demand Management." *Employee Health Benefits,* 1996, *2,* 38–44.

21. Prescott, M. "Exploring the Possibilities: Health Plans Offer Connections to Better Information Through the World Wide Web." *HMO Magazine,* 1996, *37,* 28–34.

22. Jossi, F. "A New Way to Choose a Personal Physician." *Healthplan,* 1996, *37,* 13–16.

23. McCormack, J. "Moving Beyond Billboards." *Health Data Management,* 1997, *5,* 132–134.

24. Osteraa, L., and Kelliher, M. "Appointment Scheduling." In M. McDougall and T. A. Matson (eds.), *Information Systems for Ambulatory Care.* Chicago: American Hospital Publishing, 1990.

25. Straub, K. "Right on Schedule? Demand for Enterprise-Wide Scheduling Solutions Grows." *Health Management Technology,* 1997, *18,* 32–34.

26. Coffey, R. J., and others. "Computerized Clinic Scheduling System at the University of Michigan Medical Center." *Journal of the Society for Health Systems,* 1997, *2,* 81–89.

27. Onder, L. A., and Kaatz, T. "Optimizing Resources and Access Improvement Through Balanced Scheduling in a Group Practice Setting." *NAHAM Management Journal,* Fall 1995, pp. 12–29.

28. Mead, A., Powell, D. J., and Sevilla, C. "Automated Outpatient Scheduling: A Step Toward the Integrated Delivery System." *Healthcare Information Management,* 1996, *10,* 11–21.

29. Morrissey, J. "System Simplifies Scheduling Maze." *Modern Healthcare,* 1996, *26*(19), 66–70.

30. Morrissey, J. "Machines Need to Know the Rules." *Modern Healthcare,* 1996, *26*(19), 62.

31. White, E. "Bringing Scheduling to the Enterprise." *Healthcare Informatics,* 1996, *13,* 24–30.

32. Anonymous. "Outpatient Redesign Boosts Efficiency." *Outpatient Benchmarks,* 1996, *2,* 4–66.

33. Matheson, P. A., and Fallon, L. F. "Nurse Telephone Screening of New Medicare HMO Members: A Pilot Program." *HMO Practice,* 1996, *9,* 14–18.

34. Bedeian, K., Hively, J. M., Gerstman, B. B., and Dhanoa, D. "Decreasing the Number of Recheck Appointments for an Urgent Care Clinic by Using Telephoned Follow-Up Care by Nurses." *HMO Practice,* 1996, *10,* 44–45.

35. Wasson, J., and others. "Telephone Care as a Substitute for Routine Clinic Follow-Up." *Journal of the American Medical Association,* 1992, *267,* 1788–1793.

36. Mosser, G. "Clinical Process Improvement: Engage First, Measure Later." *Quality Management in Health Care,* 1996, *4,* 11–20.

37. Magnusson, A. R., and others. "Follow-up Compliance After Emergency Department Evaluation." *Annals of Emergency Medicine,* 1993, *22,* 560–567.

38. Braly, D. "Enterprise-Wide Scheduling: Do You Need It?" *Health Management Technology,* 1996, *17,* 32–34.

CHAPTER FOUR

ACCESS TO CARE: INFORMATION MANAGEMENT CHALLENGES

Jane Metzger and Marty Geisler

This chapter focuses on the information management challenges of the new models for access to care that were described in Chapter Three and examines how these translate into system requirements. Implementing any of the emerging models requires, at a minimum, a new standard application for enterprise scheduling. The systems and support requirements become increasingly complex as more components are incorporated into the process. The chapter first presents the individual components, such as care scheduling, then the requirements for end-user integration. It concludes with a discussion of the information management challenges posed by requirements for performance measurement and the need to ensure the security and confidentiality of patient information.

The Process Components

As discussed in Chapter Three, emerging models for access to care bring together (and typically centralize) a number of previously separate functions. Traditional activities such as care scheduling and patient registration remain, as do the information requirements for these functions. In new process models, however, these activities are conducted in a uniform manner (or close to it) across the enterprise. The following discussion focuses on the information management challenges that result from centralizing and integrating old functions and introducing new ones.

Care Scheduling

Several features of the new models for access to care cannot be made operational without information system support.

Centralized Scheduling. Some of the information management challenges for care scheduling result from centralization of telephone access to appointment scheduling. In the old process, scheduling was performed in individual service areas by staff who became expert in the complex requirements for their services and providers. In contrast, a centralized staff of service representatives booking appointments for a broad range of services and settings must manage a far greater level of complexity. Primary care is very different from specialist physician services, and many individual radiology and other imaging procedures have specific requirements. New models often include physical therapy, and some also integrate scheduling for the operating room and hospital admissions. Each of these services has its own set of unique scheduling challenges.

Service representatives can do the right thing consistently for each caller and each appointment only if they are assisted in matching customer service requests with the appropriate service, in capturing the appropriate information for each scheduled service (in many cases, equivalent to the information on an order), and in asking all questions appropriately and providing necessary information and instructions. System requirements to provide these capabilities include the ability to match service requests by problem or diagnosis, and extensive scripting of the service representative's interaction with the patient.

New models are not totally centralized, however, so another core requirement is the ability to schedule appointments simultaneously from centralized and individual service areas and to control what types of appointments can be booked in either mode. Some process models restrict centralized or local appointment booking to specific users or designated schedule blocks, appointment types, or appointments. For example, triage nurses may be the only users who are allowed to book appointments in urgent care, or staff from primary care clinics may be able to book referral appointments in specialty practices only during designated blocks of time. User access must be customizable to this level of control to accommodate the variations in policies and procedures.

Complex Scheduling. An important business objective for new process models is to enable customers to schedule multiple appointments with one telephone call. Making it possible for service representatives to provide this service requires making the appointment scheduling process efficient. Customer convenience, in terms of minimizing visits to obtain care and the amount of time it takes to receive services, is also important. Another universal business objective is to improve resource utilization by minimizing the need to cancel or reschedule services because of scheduling conflicts or other contraindications. Accomplishing this requires up-front identification of potential conflicts during the appointment-scheduling process, which makes each appointment-scheduling transaction complex.

Many callers who seek to schedule hospital-based services need appointments for a set of coordinated preparatory services that must be completed prior to a hospital admission or scheduled procedure. To perform these functions, service representatives must be able to call up standard sets of services and book coordinated appointments. Service or procedure sets are akin to order sets used for electronic order entry. Keeping the set identified as a set facilitates rescheduling and canceling appointments. When combined with rules-based decision support, a change affecting any one service in the set can trigger a reminder or notification to review the other services. (This capability helps the IDN avoid a major cause of last-minute cancellations and patient no-shows.)

Rules-based decision support can improve the process in additional ways by factoring considerations into the scheduling transaction that service representatives could never accomplish independently. For example, they can

- Check for appointment conflicts, proper sequencing of procedures, and interactions of drugs or contrast media, or other contraindications

- Incorporate patient transit times into coordinated scheduling of multiple services

- Check for opportunities to coordinate scheduling with other appointments for the patient or the patient's family members

- Respect patient eligibility and payer coverage rules in appointments offered (covered services, approved providers)

- Check for compliance with enterprise appointment access standards (time lag to available appointment) so that alternatives can be explored when necessary

Centralized models virtually always require the first two services—conflict checking and patient transit time—to meet basic business objectives. The remaining items are usually on wish lists for the future because of the limitations of current scheduling products.

Patient Support. Preparing patients with information and assistance in advance of the encounter is important in virtually all new access models. At the most basic level, this includes coordinated reminders, either by telephone or mail, and service-related instructions and directions. Customizing these into an agenda for care for patients with multiple services improves customer service. Features may include directions for driving and parking, information on the sequence and timing of services, and explanations about what to expect and how to prepare (for example, dietary restrictions or suitable clothing).

Although not broadly implemented today, faxes and the Internet will soon be common vehicles for patients and provider organizations to communicate service-related information. These will undoubtedly be used for patient reminders and service-related instructions. A number of organizations plan to facilitate patient scheduling of appointments via the Internet.[1] Interactive voice response is being used for patient reminders,[2,3] and patient messaging and appointment scheduling via this mode are likely in the future.

Managing Appointment Access. Virtually all organizations set target performance levels for appointment access and manage scheduling and resources to consistently meet them. Several capabilities are required to provide the necessary information. Supervisors need easy access to information on appointment availability on an ad hoc basis so they can respond to demands for services with changes in appointment mix and service resources.

Understanding patients' experience in attempting to obtain appointments requires good information about demand for services. As part of this, the ability to track unsatisfied service requests is critical; without this information the organization has no chance of understanding the true demand for services or of notifying providers when a caller request is not met. Ideally all such calls are documented, including the type of appointment and service provider requested, and the information is incorporated into management reports. Unfortunately, most current scheduling products do not capture information on unfulfilled requests for services. Some organizations attempt to have service representatives record this information; an interim solution in call centers is to use call management software to log these calls.

Cross-Continuum Support. The need to address services across the continuum of care produces other challenges for those providers operating new access models. Basically, the enterprise scheduling application must provide support for all of the legacy scheduling applications it replaces, as well as fill in gaps where scheduling was manual. Some of the enterprise scheduling products on the market evolved from a prior inpatient- or ambulatory-focused product, and some do not yet have the ability to handle the full range of services found in many enterprise models. Project managers and staff involved with vendor evaluations recommend the following as good indicators of a truly broad-spectrum application design:

- Scheduling linked with order entry (especially inpatient order entry)
- Ambulatory medical record tracking for scheduled appointments, including tools for managing record transfers across sites and medical record rooms in the enterprise
- Ease of booking, rebooking, and canceling a series of appointments (for example, for physical or radiation therapy)
- Service scheduling and booking of services that require a room, one or more pieces of equipment, and one or more providers or support staff (for example, nuclear medicine)

Even if the initial rollout is limited to hospital-based or ambulatory care services, an organization will preserve future flexibility if its scheduling application can handle the full range of scheduling requirements for cross-continuum services.

Integrated Patient Accounting

Incorporating the front-end functions of patient accounting or billing into the access process requires that staff accomplish these tasks in real time. Some business objectives cannot be fully met without real-time data exchange with payers.

Unified Registration. In most models, service representatives in centralized scheduling or access centers complete and update patient registrations and insurance information. Accomplishing this efficiently requires accessing one set of registration information for each patient and incorporating any updates into the information to be used in downstream processes such as encounter management and billing. In some models the task is split, and new registrations or completed miniregistrations are referred to staff who specialize in this function (a registration unit). Full registration can also be delayed for some patients who are unable or unwilling to spend the time on the telephone to supply all of the necessary information. Both practices require the ability to track registration status for each patient with scheduled services and to manage open registration tasks until they are completed.

Insurance Verification. Real-time insurance verification is a part of every new access model and a sticking point for every implementation. It avoids the rework and surprises that can arise when verification occurs later or when unresolved insurance-related issues result in denied claims or bills. Organizations identified in our research are generally able to accommodate more on-line verification with payers than they have achieved. The bottleneck appears to be primarily on the payer side, because many are reluctant or unable to make eligibility information available on-line.

Because of this situation, staff in many organizations devise work-arounds that they hope to phase out over time. In the meantime, however, work-arounds bring their own information management challenges. A typical work-around is to refer records of patients with newly scheduled services to a group of staff who call insurers to verify patient eligibility. Accomplishing this requires workflow management to track each patient until insurance has been verified or the patient has been notified. Because the process is so labor-intensive, many organizations choose to focus verification on types of services in which the financial risk is greatest, and to exclude patients whose insurance has been recently verified. Rules-based decision support is required to incorporate these considerations into the verification task.

Patient Account Management. Some new models for access to care incorporate functions previously performed in the billing office or at check-in. The functions themselves are familiar, but they are now performed in conjunction with scheduling rather than with encounter management or billing. In some organizations, service representatives offer patients the ability to prepay co-payments and other service fees. Others advise the patient of the full cost of a course of treatment (for example, a series of physical therapy visits) in advance or use the opportunity to discuss outstanding account balances and perhaps even perform financial counseling. All of these services require that the service representative have access to up-to-date information on account balances and be able to post payments to patient accounts. If patient accounts with balances in excess of a predetermined amount are to be flagged, rules-based decision support is required as well.

Telephone Response

Information system support is required for managing the telephone service function and providing a high level of customer service.

Managing a Call Center. Organizations implementing centralized telephone access are emulating the call centers operated in many other service industries.[4, 5, 6, 7] In health care organizations that operate their own health plans, call centers may be in place for member services. For most health care providers, however, call centers are a new venture. In addition to advanced telecommunications, information management is key to meeting business objectives for improving the efficiency of telephone response to customer calls.

A core information requirement for supervisors is immediate access to concurrent data on call volume, calls waiting, and other indicators used to manage call response. This obviously must come from the telecommunications system and be available both within the call center and in management offices so that managers and supervisors can easily monitor current status.

Call Logging. Logging every call is important for several reasons. It provides necessary information for call tracking and completion management (for those calls requiring a call-back or follow-up) and important information on the number and types of calls, which facilitates supervision of service representatives and call center management. When call logging includes call subject and outcome, it provides an important window on the state of the business that can highlight areas for operations improvement.[4, 7] For example, numerous calls from patients with questions about benefits can point out the need for better member orientation and education, and frequent calls to change primary care physician (PCP) assignments may signal service-related problems in individual practices or inadequate information on staffing and hours of service in the materials available to new members.

Customer Service. One-stop shopping and first-call resolution are universal business objectives for call centers in any industry and are included in the objectives for telephone response in new access models for health care. These objectives are separate but interrelated. One-stop shopping means that the customer can accomplish multiple service objectives in one call. First-call resolution means that as often as possible all of a customer's needs are fully addressed during the call (the patient is not required to call elsewhere and no follow-up call to the patient is necessary).

To accomplish this level of customer service, the service representative must have access to caller-specific information, enterprise information resources, and business applications to resolve the caller's issue. For access call centers in health care, basic caller-specific information includes patient identification, demographics, and information on their insurance or managed care plan. This information provides the foundation for serving the customer and keeping track of customer interactions. For restricted-access services such as triage, it also establishes patient eligibility for the service in some cases. Depending on the subject of the call, basic information may include caller history. Computer-telephone integration, combined with automatic telephone number identification or caller entry of identification number via telephone keypad, can speed retrieval of caller-specific information. This allows the service representatives to view information about callers as they answer the call and even to greet the caller by name.

Customers often call telephone access centers to obtain simple information such as driving directions or hours of service. Some callers need assistance in identifying a physician who provides the service they seek. In access to care models, call management often requires that service representatives have up-to-date information on health plan benefits. Staff in call centers need access to all of these types of information, with an index or search capability to locate the information they need quickly.

The business applications that are needed depend on the functions integrated into the telephone access center. These are crucial to customer service goals and efficiency. For example, if the patient requests a new PCP, this should be recorded during the call, eliminating the need for the service representative to call or send a message to another department for subsequent recording in the managed care application. Likewise, the call outcome may include sending service-related instructions and information to the patient or posting a co-payment to the patient's account; if these tasks are handed off to another department rather than set in motion at the conclusion of the call, delays and task repetition are likely to result. The more transactions that service representatives can complete on-line, the greater will be the downstream benefits.

Ideal Patient Encounter

Many of the desired improvements in the patient encounter cannot be achieved without new common applications and, in some cases, totally new functions.

One-Stop Check-In. Business objectives for improving the patient encounter focus primarily on making the care experience efficient and pleasant for the patient. This involves streamlining the steps in the process. The patient encounter begins with on-site registration (check-in). Many emerging access to care models include one-stop patient registration, even for patients who receive multiple services. This is possible only if the service areas in the local site share a common registration process (and a common registration application). One-stop check-in is generally easier to accomplish in an ambulatory care site than in a hospital or medical center, where a broader variety of service types is involved.

One-stop registration should accomplish reimbursement-related activities such as checking identification cards, resolving any insurance-related loose ends, and collecting co-payments. Ideally it also captures patient arrival time and communicates this information to all service areas in which the patient has an appointment.

Managing Patient Encounters. Another objective for the patient encounter is to ensure that the patient's time is spent receiving service rather than waiting to receive it. Reducing patient waits and delays requires that both support staff and providers be able to track where patients are and who should be seen next. Especially in physician offices, information for patient tracking is usually limited to patient check-in time, and only staff working at the front desk are able to view it. This is obviously of limited value beyond the first phase of the encounter.

Providing information for staff at practice sites to monitor and proactively manage patient flow requires two types of support: information on patient location and waiting status for staff who are responsible for guiding patients to examination rooms ("rooming"), and information for individual providers concerning location, service sequencing, and waiting status of their patients. Because the information constantly changes, the ideal solution is akin to an electronic display that functions like the familiar "grease board" on acute care units. The view for practice staff would include all patients in a given area, whereas individual providers would see only their patients. (Though visible to staff, the information should not be visible to patients or visitors, to protect patient confidentiality.)

Capturing the start and end times of the clinician interaction is critical to managing patient flow. This information is also required as input to reengineering visit times to correspond with the amount of time actually required for the type of encounter (another strategy for reducing patient waits and delays). Some organizations have providers record times for research or management purposes, but this is impractical in the busy ambulatory setting. Other organizations have considered using sensing or card-swipe technology to detect when providers enter and leave examination rooms. To be useful, this information must be integrated in some way with data on patient scheduling and exam room assignment, and the technology is probably more feasible in new facilities. The most natural way to capture information on clinician–patient interaction time is as a by-product of the provider signing on to, and then signing off from, a patient care system in the exam room. The same approach can capture interaction times when providers obtain vital signs and perform other activities as part of the encounter. Further advances and more widespread implementation of point-of-service information technology in the ambulatory setting will be required before it is feasible to capture such information routinely.

Another target for improving the encounter is anticipation of patient needs so that the patient feels expected and welcome. Some of this revolves around special needs, such as for transportation or foreign language interpreters. Some organizations, however, also flag patients with hearing disabilities or patients who may have difficulty finding their way around large facilities. Addressing unique patient needs requires, at a minimum, capturing information on needs as part of registration or scheduling and communicating it to service sites. When transportation or other assistance is needed, the ability to generate work lists is also useful.

Managed Care and Member Services

Once an organization provides a significant volume of at-risk care, integrating membership and plan-related functions into the access process becomes desirable. Accomplishing this efficiently, from the standpoint of both the customer and the health care system, requires the access center staff to use the necessary applications in real time.

Member Services. Organizations that provide at-risk care typically incorporate some managed care payer-related functions into the new access process. These functions can include selection or change of PCP, requests for replacement identification cards, or filing of complaints about services or other issues. In health care systems that operate their own health plan, enrollment- and claims-related inquiries may also be included to permit one-call customer access to the system.

To meet customer service goals, service representatives in enterprise access centers need member-specific information from various databases. This always includes patient eligibility and health plan benefits but may also include patient enrollment status and claims processing. When updates occur to PCP designation or a new member identification card must be sent, service representatives also complete (or initiate) certain transactions to avoid an inefficient multistep process or hand-off to another department.

Synchronizing information such as current PCP in scheduling and managed care databases requires bidirectional updates, because the information is often maintained in both locations and updates can be entered at either one. The inability to achieve data synchronization leads to additional tasks for staff or ongoing problems with physician panel and capitation management.

Health plans were early adopters of Web sites for members to accomplish several kinds of transactions. The most typical interactive tasks include reviewing benefits information, requesting an identification card, and selecting or changing a PCP.[8, 9]

New-Member Orientation. Many organizations seek to welcome and connect with new members by calling them to ensure that they understand how and where to seek care and information and to assist with PCP selection. Both of these services require identifying the patients to be contacted from enrollment information or from a subpopulation such as Medicare enrollees. Calls can be accomplished most efficiently with call-out lists and other workflow management tools that organize the activity and track completion and outcome of calls. (In organizations that accomplish new-member risk screening by telephone, this is ideally integrated with other orientation activities so that new members are contacted only once.)

Triage

Integrating triage has several prerequisites, but computer support for triage protocols or algorithms is essential. Shared access to electronic patient information and messaging are key to continuity of care.

Triage Protocols. Triage is always guided by evidence-based protocols or algorithms.[10, 11] Many organizations purchase triage software from a vendor, because the development costs are enormous and continual updating is mandatory to reflect changes in practice. Triage nurses must be able to access the appropriate protocol or algorithm based on symptom, problem, or diagnosis and patient group (usually age categories and sex). Documenting the patient interaction and the outcome of the call, critical for both medicolegal reasons and continuity of care, is also standard practice.

Patient Information Access. The triage process can be supported with patient information at three levels:

1. All patient-specific information must be obtained from the patient during triage (although some triage applications permit the triage nurse to view notes from previously documented triage sessions).
2. The triage nurse can view historical patient clinical information during the interaction but must enter any new patient-provided information.
3. Relevant electronic patient history information can be incorporated automatically into the triage protocol or algorithm so that the triage nurse need only confirm completeness and enter new information.

Our research identified examples of the first and second levels. As integrated triage is implemented in organizations with electronic medical records, the automatic incorporation of patient data into triage protocols or algorithms will be the logical next step. This will speed the interaction and give patients and providers increased confidence that all relevant information is available and being used. In the area of medications, either level two or level three support will be extremely useful, because many patients have difficulty remembering the names and dosages of the medications they take, and this information is frequently relevant to triage.

Continuity of Care. Provider access to triage notes is important for continuity of care. Timeliness of the communication is especially important when the patient will be communicating with the provider soon after triage, either in person or by telephone. Direct provider access to triage notes can be accomplished through electronic messaging or a shared patient care information system (in which triage notes are incorporated into the patient's electronic health history). Because most organizations still lack such a system, faxing triage notes to the physician practice or location where the patient's medical record resides is common practice.

Many organizations distribute standard patient education materials to complement triage as part of a larger demand management program. Continuity of care is enhanced when these materials are integrated into the triage process. This can be accomplished in different ways, for example, through

- Patient direct access to standard educational materials (independent access through keypad selections on the telephone or interactive voice response)
- Patient access to standard educational materials offered by a service representative or triage nurse (mailed out following the call)
- Triage nurse access to standard educational materials issued by the organization for use during patient interactions (both patient and provider looking at and discussing the same material)
- Triage nurse access during telephone conversations to patient-specific customized materials already provided to the patient (for example, access to materials given at discharge from the emergency department or acute care) to reinforce teaching or answer patient questions

Our research found examples of the first two approaches and future plans to incorporate the second two approaches as soon as information systems permit. Providing patient-accessible educational materials on health-related topics was one of the earliest features of health plan and health care system Web sites.[12, 13, 14, 15, 16]

Referrals. Patients, clinicians, and the health care system all welcome improvements in referral management. Consequently, new process models may include activities such as the following to streamline and simplify referral processing:

Service representatives and triage nurses record patient requests.

Requests are electronically routed to PCPs for review.

Approved requests are routed back to the scheduling center, where staff notify the patient and make necessary arrangements.

These steps require capabilities for documenting patient requests and electronic messaging between clinicians and access center staff.

Rules-based decision support can help staff directly process patient-requested referrals in accordance with health plan rules (especially useful for services that do not require a referral). Ideally, advanced patient care systems will provide tools for authorizing patient referrals in cases in which appropriateness criteria are clearly met.[17, 18] Some current algorithm-based triage applications include a capability for recommending immediate referral to a specialist or to acute care as an outcome of triage.

Clinical Outreach

Clinical outreach can be implemented only with sophisticated support to the care management functions and real-time communication between physicians and providers in clinics and other practice sites.

Provider-Requested Outreach. Although our research found fewer examples of clinical outreach than of triage, some organizations are taking advantage of the presence of triage nurses in the access center to make outgoing calls to patients as part of care management. The most common type of call is requested by a provider—sometimes by the patient's primary physician or primary care case manager, sometimes by a triage nurse as a follow-up to an earlier triage call.

To communicate such requests, PCPs, primary care case managers, triage nurses, and other providers must be able to specify patient, subject, and timing for telephone outreach. Triage software often permits the triage nurse to place a reminder for a follow-up call. To communicate requests from other providers, it is ideal to combine electronic messaging with workflow management to create call-out work lists. Return messaging to physicians or case managers can notify them of call completions and outcomes.

Protocol-Based Outreach. Examples of protocol-based outreach include callback to patients referred to an emergency room after triage, patients recently discharged from acute care, and patients who have recently had ambulatory surgery. Some outreach programs seek to replace the need for patients to do their own follow-up. For example, certain types of diagnostic procedures can be flagged for patient notification by telephone call (such as results of throat cultures and other designated procedures).

Rules-based decision support is required to flag patients for protocol-based outreach. On their end, triage nurses require sufficient information on the clinical situation to make each call, workflow management functions (such as work lists, patient contact information, task tracking), and the ability to document patient interactions (see the scenarios in Chapter Five for examples).

Member Risk Screening. As discussed in Chapter Six, integrated care systems that provide at-risk care are implementing risk screening of new members to identify candidates for special care management programs. Risk-screening is often combined with new-member outreach, although we found examples of these both singly and in combination. Integrating new-member call-out into access center operations for this purpose requires the ability to identify new members (sometimes a subgroup based on age or other characteristics) and to administer and record responses to a standard risk-screening instrument. Real-time analysis of patient responses and risk stratification based on the resulting score can enable the triage nurse to initiate protocol-based responses during the initial telephone interaction (see Chapter Eight for an example scenario).

Supporting Cross-Functional Roles

New models for centralized access integrate many of the functions that were previously performed in different areas and departments, so each staff member must be able to perform a range of tasks. The most cross-functional roles for health system staff are in enterprise scheduling or access centers where patients call for a range of services and information. In models for both centralized enterprise scheduling and access to care, service representatives handle incoming calls. The addition of triage and other care-management initiatives brings triage nurses into the access center. Each call can potentially involve any combination and sequence of activities for these two roles, as summarized in Figures 4.1 and 4.2.

No vendor offers a single software application or set of integrated applications that can support all of the tasks required. (Project managers in health systems that have implemented enterprise scheduling caution that vendor claims about the integration of their products are currently inflated.) For the staff in call centers, handling each call efficiently requires accessing and capturing information in a variety of applications. For the service representative this can involve registration, scheduling, billing, managed care enrollment and member services, and

FIGURE 4.1. POTENTIAL USER ACTIVITIES FOR ANY TELEPHONE CALL TO SERVICE REPRESENTATIVES IN CENTRALIZED TELEPHONE ACCESS CENTERS.

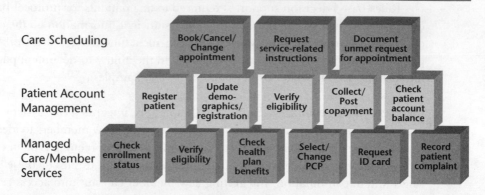

complaint management. The triage nurse must also have access to a triage application, referral processing, a patient care system, or electronic messaging, depending on the care management initiatives implemented. Seamless support requires single-user sign-on and patient identification, and the ability to accomplish tasks in any sequence once the caller has been identified.

Performance Monitoring

As discussed in Chapter Three, new enterprise scheduling or access processes are managed to meet enterprise performance standards. This approach is consistent with experience and practice in other service industries in which performance standards play a key role in both process redesign and operations management.

Table 4.1 presents common performance measures for each process component. In the case examples identified in our research, the current focus is primarily on scheduling and telephone access, which are major areas of patient dissatisfaction and targets of report card initiatives such as Health Plan Employer Data Information Set (HEDIS).[19] For many health care systems, business objectives relating to patient account and encounter management are also major drivers in the design. For other components, few measures are in use today (often because of the difficulty of assembling the necessary information). The measures shown relate to typical business objectives.

Performance information for telephone access comes from the telecommunications system and contact management software. Measures relating to call

FIGURE 4.2. POTENTIAL USER ACTIVITIES FOR ANY TELEPHONE CALL TO TRIAGE NURSES IN A CENTRALIZED TELEPHONE ACCESS CENTER.

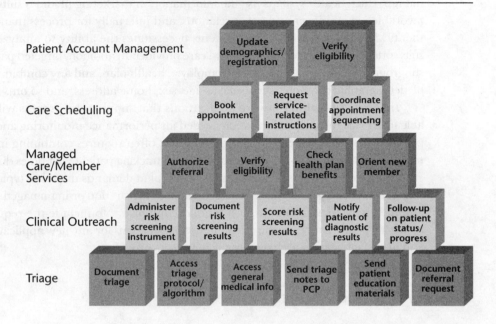

pick-up time and call abandonment must be available on a minute-by-minute basis for use by supervisors in the call center, as well as for analyzing trends in call volume by day of the week and month. This information is critical for managing call center staffing to meet performance standards consistently. Productivity (call volume, first-call resolution) of individual service representatives provides one view of their performance. Supervisors typically complement this by monitoring a sample of calls and providing coaching on quality of service and data capture.

Health systems incorporate questions about access into virtually every patient survey. Some surveys that specifically target the telephone or encounter experience are distributed (or administered by telephone) periodically to a sample of patients with recent service experience. Other surveys about patient perceptions of quality and service are distributed more broadly.[20]

The National Committee on Quality Assurance (NCQA) requires reporting on patient satisfaction with telephone and appointment access as part of annual member surveys in accredited managed care organizations. NCQA's measures (HEDIS) are now required by the Health Care Financing Administration for any health plans that cover Medicare or Medicaid patients.[21] Many health systems must respond to additional report card initiatives, sponsored by groups such as business coalitions, that include access-related information. In addition to external reporting, health systems use the information in marketing (if the results are favorable), in employer and payer relations, and internally for process management. Meeting all of these requirements necessitates the ability to analyze results sorted by care site, care setting, and care provider. In addition, targeted patient subgroups include payer type, payer, employer, health plan, and any combination of demographic characteristics (such as age, sex, home address, and so on).

In many cases, the software applications that support the process will be able to provide the basic information needed for performance monitoring and reporting. Analyzing patient subgroups, however, often requires combining information from different applications. For example, tracking patient wait times during encounters for members of a particular health plan demands data that typically reside in scheduling, encounter management, and registration or in managed care and membership applications. It is therefore important to include the requirements for performance management in the specifications for any new applications and in the application architecture for the access process.

Security Considerations

New enterprise registration, scheduling, and other applications integrate information about patient health care services much more broadly than the local legacy applications they replace. In addition, virtually all process models include decentralized information access, as well as some local scheduling (that is, local booking of appointments for follow-up care). This means that many more people have access to more comprehensive information about patient appointments and encounters using this system than they did using the fragmented processes that the system replaced.

Enterprisewide scheduling is usually the first patient care application implemented across sites and settings and thus can represent a health care system's first encounter with the challenges of ensuring security and patient confidentiality on the enterprise scale. Our research identified some health systems that intend to allow direct scheduling of appointments by office staff in affiliated (as opposed to owned or tightly integrated) community physician practices. Giving users at these sites electronic access to scheduling will further add to the challenges of ensuring patient confidentiality and controlling access.

Appointment information has traditionally been viewed as administrative information. However, it clearly meets the definition for patient-identifiable

TABLE 4.1. TYPICAL PERFORMANCE METRICS
FOR NEW ACCESS-TO-CARE MODELS.

Care Scheduling	• Next available appointment • Patients on wait list • Calls to obtain appointment • Satisfaction with access • Appointments canceled by health system • Referral booking time • Unmet requests for appointment
Telephone Response	• Call abandonment • Call pick-up time • Satisfaction with telephone response • Efficiency of resolution of reason for call (first-call resolution) • Calls meeting customer service standards
BILL $ **Patient Account Management**	• Patients scheduled without insurance verification • Patient co-pays collected • Patients seen without insurance verification • Payment denials • Days in receivable • Patients receiving financial counseling
Health System MEMBER 123-468 **Managed Care/Membership**	• Members without PCP designated • Lag time: enrollment to orientation • Patients scheduled without eligibility verification • Lag time: referral request to authorization • Member issues/complaints (by type)
Ideal Patient Encounter	• Patient wait from check-in • Patient wait time during encounter • Encounters rescheduled due to inadequate preparation • No-shows • Satisfaction with service
Triage	• Calls by reason/outcome (by type) • ED visits • Urgent care visits • Calls with change in outcome (seeking care) • Satisfaction with triage (provider and patient) • Patients accessing educational materials
Clinical Outreach	• Completion of new member screening • Lag time: enrollment to screening • Completion of protocol-based follow-up • Satisfaction (patients and providers)

information "relating to the provision of health care services to an individual"[22] and must be afforded the same safeguards and protections as clinical documentation.

Managing security and confidentiality requires an enterprise security management program that incorporates technology such as access controls and audit trails, as well as procedures for education, monitoring, and enforcement.[23] An important first step is establishing a process for setting and enforcing organizational policies and procedures.

We have not identified many examples of new enterprise scheduling models that incorporate behavioral health services, and the challenge of providing added security for the information captured is undoubtedly a factor—access-to-care processes will inevitably capture information concerning employees of the health care organization and celebrity patients. Both the technology for managing information access and the policies and procedures in place will need to incorporate additional measures for preserving patient confidentiality in these cases. Clearly, audit trails on information retrieval and the ability to exclude behavioral health data from appointment and encounter histories will be required. Access controls will have to incorporate "need to know" rules or rules regarding user identification and location (for example, viewable only in a behavioral health service area).

Several organizations with an enterprise security management program that features technical safeguards such as audit trails are including behavioral health services in appointment and encounter histories.[24, 25] However, most organizations appear to be awaiting clarification of responsibilities and acceptable protections before including sensitive services in new access models.

Conclusions

Health systems that are implementing new models for enterprise scheduling and access to care face significant information management challenges. The processes simply cannot be implemented without advanced information and telecommunications technology.

In the cases examined in our research, this has meant implementing new common applications for enterprise scheduling and other functions that must be integrated into the new process. Centralized telephone access is a core feature of new process models, and call center staff perform multiple functions. Making their work efficient and effective requires seamless integration of multiple software applications on the desktop.

Performance measurement and patient confidentiality and security are additional requirements that must be addressed by the organization's information management strategy and systems.

Chapter Five combines the information support discussed in this chapter with the process for enterprise access to care discussed in Chapter Three to illustrate how key participants such as triage nurses and primary care physicians interact with information technology as they perform their roles in the new process.

Notes

1. Sunquist, J. "The Health Village Pilot: Tuning Up an Internet Solution." *Health Management Technology*, 1997, *11*, 38–40.
2. Wulf, S., and LeVine, P. "Automated Patient Monitoring Using Interactive Voice Response Technology." *Healthcare Innovations*, 1997, *7*, 20–22.
3. Balas, E. A., and others. "Electronic Communication with Patients: Evaluation of Distance Medicine Technology." *Journal of the American Medical Association*, 1997, *278*, 152–159.
4. Nash, J. "Fast Fone Farms, Fat Profits." *CIO*, 1997, *10* (1), 40–52.
5. Cooperstein, D. "Click Here for an Agent." *CIO*, 1997, *10* (1), 36–37.
6. "An Exchange of Knowledge Among Leading Practitioners in Customer Management." Cambridge, Mass.: Arthur D. Little, 1994, pp. 3–6.
7. Rappaport, D. M. "The Press for More Options." *CIO*, 1997, *10*, 30–34.
8. Prescott, M. "Exploring the Possibilities: Health Plans Offer Connections to Better Information Through the Worldwide Web." *HMO Magazine*, 1996, *37*, 28–34.
9. McCormack, J. "Moving Beyond Billboards." *Health Data Management*, 1997, *5*, 132–134.
10. Morrisey, J. "On Call: Health Systems' Sophisticated Telephone Triage Center Wins Popularity with Patients and Physicians." *Modern Healthcare*, 1997, *27*, 72–80.
11. Prescott, M. "A Friendly Voice in the Night." *Healthplan*, 1996, *37*, 47–53.
12. Hovey, J. V. "The Potential: Powerful Changes Are Afoot as Health Plans Use Internet Technology for Customer Service." *Healthplan*, 1997, *38*, 41–47.
13. Jaklevic, M. C. "Internet Technology Moves to Patient-Care Front Lines." *Modern Healthcare*, 1997, *3* (11), 47–50.
14. Brown, E. "Where to Find Medical Advice on the Web." *Fortune*, 1997, *3* (17), 62.
15. Chin, T. L. "Patient Education at the Crossroads." *Health Data Management*, 1997, *5*, 106.
16. Mullich, J. "Intranet Gives HMO a Shot in the Arm." *PC Week*, 1997, *14*, 27.
17. Einbinder, J. S., Klein, D. A., and Safran, C. S. "Making Effective Referrals: A Knowledge-Management Approach." In D. R. Masys (ed.), *Journal of the American Medical Informatics Association Fall Proceedings 1997*. Philadelphia: Belfus, pp. 330–334.
18. Ladenson, P. W., Kelleher, G., Murphy, S., and Overhage, J. M. "Clinical Referrals: The Two-Edged Sword of Health Care." Panel discussion during the Journal of the American Medical Informatics Association fall conference, Nashville, Tennessee, Nov. 1997.
19. Anonymous. "The HEDIS Domains and Descriptions of the Measures." *In Health Plan Employer Data and Information Set and Users' Manual, Version 3.0*. Washington, D.C.: National Council on Quality Assurance, 1997, pp. 29–70.
20. Tarlov, A. R. *National Library of Healthcare Indicators: Health Plan and Network Edition*. Oakbrook Terrace, Ill.: Joint Commission on Accreditation of Healthcare Organizations, 1997.
21. Hagland, M. "Ducks in a Row: Experts Offer Practical Advice on Critical Information Systems Strategies for Success in the Emerging World of Quality Report Cards." *Healthplan*, 1997, *38* (2), 23–25.

22. http://aspe.os.dhhs.gov/ncvhs.security.htm

23. Committee on Maintaining Privacy and Security in Health Care Applications of the National Information Infrastructure. *For the Record: Protecting Electronic Health Information.* Washington, D.C.: National Academy Press, 1997.

24. Khoury, A., Siemon, C., Mills, G., and Kalata, M. "The Medical Automated Record System of Kaiser Permanente of Ohio." In J. M. Teich (ed.), *Third Annual Nicholas E. Davies CPR Recognition Symposium.* Schaumburg, Ill.: Computer-Based Patient Record Institute, 1997, pp. 5–72.

25. Cochran, D. "Confidentiality of Computer-Based Patient Records: Consumer Perspectives." Presentation delivered at the CPRI fall meeting, Nashville, Tenn., Oct. 1997.

CHAPTER FIVE

ACCESS TO CARE: A SNAPSHOT OF THE FUTURE PROCESS

Jane Metzger, Derek Messie, and Thomas Hurley

This chapter ties together the new process models described in Chapter Three and the information requirements discussed in Chapter Four into a process scenario. The scenario uses First-Rate Health, a fictitious IDN, to illustrate one integrated care model. It includes a medical center, several community hospitals, a medical group of employed primary care and specialist physicians, skilled nursing and rehab services, and home care. First-Rate Health is located in a metropolitan market with several dominant employers that have encouraged employees to select health plans as their health insurance; it also operates in a state that offers Medicare beneficiaries a health plan option. Consequently, 70 percent of First-Rate Health's revenue is now prepaid reimbursement. It operates its own health plan, Good Health Plan, but also holds contracts with other plans to provide at-risk care.

First-Rate Health has been an integrated care system for three years and has evolved considerably from the governance structure and organization of the original individual entities that are now part of First-Rate Health. One of its first initiatives was the creation of a new front-end process for the care system called Access to Care. This process starts with the initial patient contact with First-Rate Health at enrollment or registration and includes scheduling and encounter management as well as numerous care management activities. This chapter provides a snapshot of the new access process.

Access to Care introduces some new roles for First-Rate Health staff and enhances some traditional ones. The improvements introduced in the access-to-care process are illustrated by scenarios for the roles of a service representative, a triage nurse, a patient, and a physician:

- Most patient telephone calls come into regional access centers that First-Rate Health operates in the northern and southern regions of its service area. Service representatives answer most patient calls and schedule appointments or provide necessary service information. Their tasks can also include aiding members in selecting or changing primary care physicians (PCPs), processing requests for replacement of identification cards, and other membership-related activities.
- Working alongside service representatives in the access center are triage nurses who guide patients to appropriate care using symptom-based algorithms designed expressly for this purpose. Triage nurses also answer general health-related questions.
- Patients leave messages for PCPs and request prescription renewals by calling the access center. PCPs receive messages from triage nurses and service representatives and are routinely notified of certain types of patient interactions with the access center.
- In addition to using centralized telephone access to services and information through the access center, patients can utilize the Internet to access several Web sites operated by First-Rate Health. This provides them with additional modes of communicating with their care team and the health care system, as well as the ability to obtain information about specific health conditions and health-related services.

The scenarios in this chapter follow each of these roles for a few minutes of the routine day.

First-Rate Health has invested heavily in its information technology infrastructure to support the continuum of care with seamless information access and assistance with patient management. The result, the Enterprise System, is the patient care computer system that helps First-Rate Health ensure that there is continuity of care for each patient, and it provides a single standard of care and service everywhere in its health system. (This computer system is possible with today's technology, but the scope of integrated function and extent of implementation described are futuristic.) In our example, the Enterprise System is now utilized by staff throughout the care system. The scenarios describe how staff use the computer system to accomplish many new tasks and to communicate with one another. The computer desktop for each type of participant is customized to provide easy access to the functions used by that staff member. The many applications encompassed by the system have been integrated so that users move seamlessly from one to another and the work flows efficiently.

Screen shots from this ideal system illustrate system contributions at certain points in the scenarios.

Access Center Service Representative

We join Samantha Lundeen, one of the service representatives in First-Rate Health's access center, as she picks up a call routed to her by the telecommunications system. Call routing ensures that calls are picked up within fifteen seconds by distributing the calls within the access center and preferentially routing calls for certain physician practices to Samantha's section. This allows patients to interact with the same service representatives most of the time and enables service representatives to become familiar with frequent callers. Supervisors can easily monitor the queue of calls waiting and the pick-up times. Overflow calls are routed first to another service representative in Samantha's call center and then to another access center operated by First-Rate Health in a different part of the state. This transfer is transparent to patients because service representatives everywhere have access to the Enterprise System.

The first caller, Milo Rappen, is a patient of one of First-Rate Health's PCPs. The telecommunications system in the access center has been integrated with the Enterprise System and automatically identifies callers based on the telephone number from which they are calling. As a result, the Enterprise System calls up a patient identification screen, illustrated in Figure 5.1, and displays it on Samantha's workstation as she greets Mr. Rappen. (Note that patient contact information includes Mr. Rappen's cellular telephone number, home fax, and e-mail address; First-Rate Health uses these to communicate with him according to his preferences, which are stored in the Enterprise patient directory.)

Mr. Rappen requests an acute appointment because he is experiencing an earache that is rapidly becoming more painful. Samantha selects "acute" under Appointment, and the system checks for an appointment with Dr. McAndrew, Mr. Rappen's PCP. The next available appointment is in two days, a time lag that does not meet First-Rate Health's access standards for acute appointments with PCPs (or the patient's view of how soon he needs to be seen), so Samantha requests an urgent appointment so that Mr. Rappen can be seen sooner. The system suggests an appointment with Dr. Hersch for the next day at an urgent care clinic close to Mr. Rappen's home. Mr. Rappen accepts the appointment, and because he has never been to the urgent care clinic, Samantha offers to fax directions and an appointment confirmation to his home. After Samantha documents her activities to assist Mr. Rappen, she is ready to take another call.

FIGURE 5.1. ENTERPRISE SYSTEM VIEWED BY SERVICE REPRESENTATIVE: PATIENT DEMOGRAPHICS SCREEN.

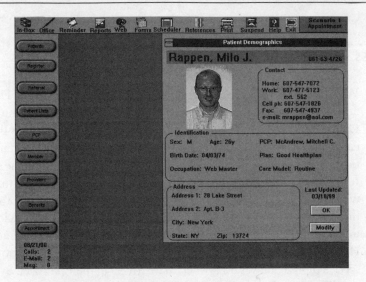

The next patient calls to request a referral to a dermatologist. First-Rate Health holds managed care contracts with so many employers and health plans that service representatives cannot possibly remember all of the detailed coverage rules (which also change frequently). The Enterprise System assists with prompts relevant to each patient's coverage and service rules. It also verifies eligibility by checking information in the managed care member database, which receives batch updates from health plans and employers each night.

Samantha confirms that the caller is Mark Stevens and enters his referral request in the system. She submits the request and is advised that his health plan does not require a referral for this type of service. She cancels the referral request and proceeds to book an appointment with a dermatologist covered by Mr. Stevens's plan. The system prompts her to advise Mr. Stevens that he will be responsible for a $10 co-payment, and he chooses to prepay by credit card. As shown in Figure 5.2, Samantha verifies his credit card information and processes the payment, which will be posted to his account in the patient accounting system.

Service representatives verify patient demographic and insurance information on a regular basis. The Enterprise System includes decision support to remind them to do so for patients whose information has not been verified during

FIGURE 5.2. ENTERPRISE SYSTEM VIEWED BY SERVICE REPRESENTATIVE: PATIENT PREPAYMENT SCREEN.

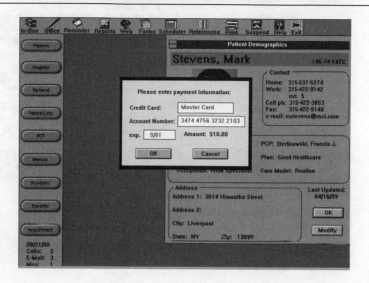

the prior sixty days. Samantha is prompted to review this information with Mark Stevens. She clicks *OK* when he indicates that no changes have occurred, and the system updates the review date. (When Mr. Stevens checks in for his appointment, he will not be asked again, because his information has recently been verified.) Mr. Stevens accepts Samantha's offer to have directions to the dermatologist's office sent to his office e-mail address.

Samantha's next call is from a referring physician practice in the community. Dr. Chesley is going to perform hip replacement surgery for Merriam Prosser, and his assistant wishes to schedule the preoperative evaluation and testing. Samantha identifies the patient in question in the Enterprise System, confirms that the operating room has been scheduled, and requests preoperative appointments. Dr. Chesley's set of standard preoperative procedures includes a chest X-ray, an EKG, a visit to the blood bank for typing and autologous blood donation, a fifteen-minute appointment with the anesthesiologist who regularly assists him, and finally, a stop in the laboratory. As shown in Figure 5.3, the system pulls up a potential series of appointments that reflect Dr. Chesley's preferences, as well as other considerations. These appointments have been selected on the basis of the decision support in the Enterprise System to accomplish all of these services in one visit to the hospital two days before surgery. The selected appointment schedule sequences

FIGURE 5.3. ENTERPRISE SYSTEM VIEWED BY SERVICE REPRESENTATIVE: SELECTED PATIENT APPOINTMENTS SCREEN.

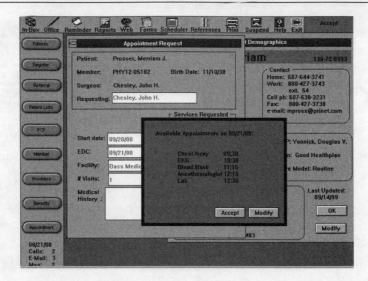

the services appropriately to avoid clinical contraindications and to allow Ms. Prosser sufficient time to walk between service locations.

First-Rate Health will send Ms. Prosser an agenda for care that includes driving and parking instructions, directions to each service area, and an explanation of what will occur in each area. The package will also include consent forms that Ms. Prosser must read and sign before her surgery. She accepts Samantha's offer to fax the paperwork to her home fax machine.

The next call is from Debra Martin, who received a reminder notice from First-Rate Health to schedule a mammogram. Samantha requests an appointment in the Enterprise System, but the next one available at the medical center is in sixty days. A system prompt reminds Samantha that this does not meet First-Rate Health's thirty-day service standard, so Samantha searches for another location, using Ms. Martin's office zip code to identify one that is convenient. Rochester Clinic, which is only a short drive away, has an open appointment in three weeks. Ms. Martin accepts the appointment and requests that directions be sent to her home. As shown in Figure 5.4, Samantha is prompted to remind Ms. Martin to wear appropriate clothing and not to use talcum powder, because that can interfere with the image quality of the mammogram.

FIGURE 5.4. ENTERPRISE SYSTEM VIEWED BY SERVICE REPRESENTATIVE: PATIENT REMINDER SCREEN.

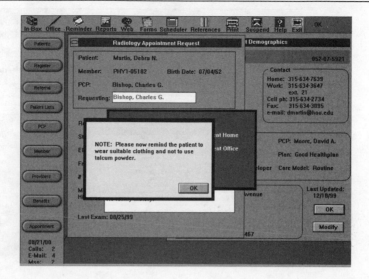

Triage Nurse

Adelle Wilder is a triage nurse who works alongside Samantha in the access center. Patients who call are given the option of speaking with a triage nurse or a service representative, or they can request prerecorded information on a variety of topics related to symptoms and general health. Patients indicate their choice by pushing the appropriate number on their telephone keypad. Samantha and other service representatives also direct calls to the triage nurse when a patient needs assistance in determining the appropriate type of health care service or has medical problems that have been targeted by First-Rate Health for telephone management.

Adelle's first caller is Wilma Rodgers, a sixty-six-year-old patient who selected the option to speak with a triage nurse when she dialed in to the access center. Because of computer-telephone integration and automated number identification, Adelle is looking at the demographics screen for Ms. Rodgers as she greets her. Ms. Rodgers starts to describe the persistent pain she is experiencing in her lower back—the reason for her call.

First-Rate Health has licensed the FirstHelp® system (U.S. patent 5471381) from Access Health, which triage nurses can consult as they obtain information from patients and use to give them care management advice. Clinical algorithms

FIGURE 5.5. ENTERPRISE SYSTEM VIEWED BY TRIAGE NURSE: SEARCH SCREEN FOR TRIAGE ALGORITHM.

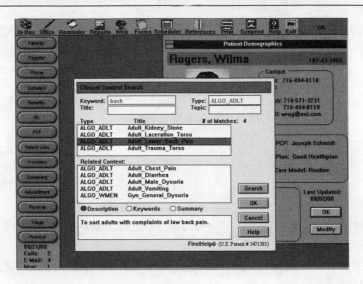

in the software guide the conversation based on patient age and sex, and in response to the answers to questions displayed on the computer screen. The purpose of guiding the questions in this way is to ensure that appropriate information on what is (and what is not) present in each situation is considered. Each of these circumstances represents a decision point in the algorithm, with appropriate branching logic based on the information obtained.

After learning that Ms. Rodgers' problem is lower back pain, Adelle uses keywords to locate the appropriate algorithm in the software, which then guides her assessment of the patient's clinical situation, as shown in Figure 5.5. For each question, Adelle is provided with a display of the clinical question, the rationale for asking it, and the question phrased in lay terms. She documents the patient's answers and can also record comments. This documentation provides coded information used to trigger rules in the triage algorithm that prompt the nurse with the next question. It also provides a complete record of the conversation and care management advice, which is then incorporated into the patient's electronic health record. Triage notes are also forwarded to the patient's PCP for review.

As Adelle guides the conversation, Ms. Rodgers explains that she is not experiencing any associated pain or pressure. Had Adelle recorded a positive answer, the triage software would have displayed any additional questions necessary to determine the appropriate care management strategy. In response to the next

FIGURE 5.6. ENTERPRISE SYSTEM VIEWED BY TRIAGE NURSE: CLINICAL CONTENT SCREEN FOR ADULT LOWER BACK PAIN.

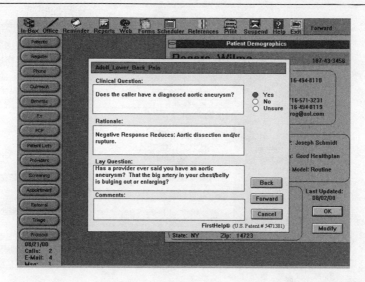

question and as shown in Figure 5.6, Ms. Rodgers indicates that she does have an aortic aneurysm, an enlargement of the aorta.

Once Adelle records this information, the next question displayed addresses symptoms that might indicate occlusion affecting a femoral artery. Adelle asks Ms. Rodgers if she has noticed anything unusual about her feet, and Ms. Rodgers replies that she has not but she does have some numbness in both legs. Based on this additional information, the algorithm displays a recommendation that the patient see her PCP within the next three days (an "early illness appointment"; see Figure 5.7).

Adelle records her agreement with the recommendation and offers to schedule the appointment. Ms. Rogers indicates, however, that she has other routine care appointments to schedule, so Adelle transfers her to a service representative. Adelle makes note of the patient's intention to seek an acute appointment with her physician. Had the conversation revealed a different history and set of symptoms, other possible algorithm recommendations would include calling for an ambulance, referring the patient to urgent care, booking a routine appointment, providing self-care instructions, or advising the patient to call his or her doctor. Care management strategies for some triage situations include immediate referral to an emergency room or to a specialist physician for consultation and treatment. When Adelle and other triage nurses preauthorize these referrals, First-Rate Health's Enterprise System sends appropriate electronic communications to the provider and the claims system.

FIGURE 5.7. ENTERPRISE SYSTEM VIEWED BY TRIAGE NURSE: ACTION LIST SCREEN.

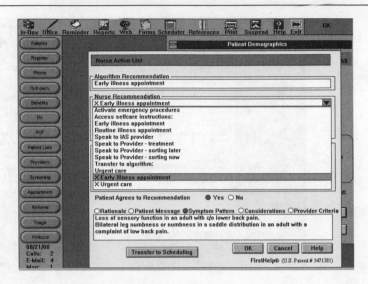

Triage nurses also perform outreach as part of several practice improvement initiatives implemented by First-Rate Health. After taking her first call, Adelle is advised by her supervisor that the call volume is light and she is taking Adelle off-line so that she can make calls to patients. To do this, Adelle clicks on the Outreach button. The system displays her work list of outreach calls for the day. These have come to her for a variety of reasons: some were prompted by rules-based decision support in First-Rate Health's Enterprise System, some were requested by a patient's PCP or primary care case manager, and some are reminders that Adelle placed in the system for herself.

Her first task is to call John McBlane, who requested the results of a recent laboratory test to determine his blood level of dilantin. (His PCP requests these tests periodically to check the dosage Mr. McBlane should be taking to control seizures.) The outreach telephone note screen is shown in Figure 5.8. Adelle reaches Mr. McBlane on her first try and explains that his test results indicate that no change in dosage will be necessary. She signs the note, which will be incorporated into Mr. McBlane's electronic medical record, with a copy forwarded to his PCP.

First-Rate Health has a policy of taking advantage of every patient interaction to schedule wellness interventions. This is made possible by the rules-based decision support and complete patient history information maintained in the Enterprise System. While still on the telephone with Mr. McBlane, Adelle receives a

FIGURE 5.8. ENTERPRISE SYSTEM VIEWED BY TRIAGE NURSE: OUTREACH TELEPHONE NOTE SCREEN.

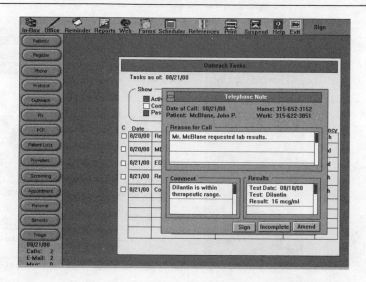

prompt to notify him that a blood pressure check and cholesterol screening are due, and she offers to schedule them. Mr. McBlane accepts the offer. The system displays his PCP's schedule for the end of the month, when a short appointment for interventions such as blood pressure checks is available. Adelle offers the time highlighted in the display and Mr. McBlane agrees. When he goes in for the appointment, the order for the cholesterol screening test will be at the laboratory, where he can stop by after he sees his PCP. The appointment is several weeks away, and Mr. McBlane requests that a routine appointment reminder be sent to him on his office e-mail, as shown in Figure 5.9.

The call volume has picked up again, and an incoming call from Suzanne Richfield is routed to Adelle. Ms. Richfield called the access center to request an appointment with her PCP because she believes she has a urinary tract infection (UTI). The service representative she spoke with explained that First-Rate Health is using a new guideline to assist patients with UTI and offered to transfer her to one of the nurses to learn more about the program.

First-Rate Health's clinical practice committee obtained the guideline from the Institute for Clinical Systems Integration in Minneapolis.[1, 2, 3] The guideline changes practices in several ways. First, after careful screening of patients, the nurse can initiate treatment without a urine culture (the culture requires the patient to come into the laboratory to provide a specimen and also incurs the cost of testing). Patients who satisfy all of the criteria in the guideline need not come

FIGURE 5.9. ENTERPRISE SYSTEM VIEWED BY TRIAGE NURSE: REMINDER DELIVERY OPTIONS SCREEN.

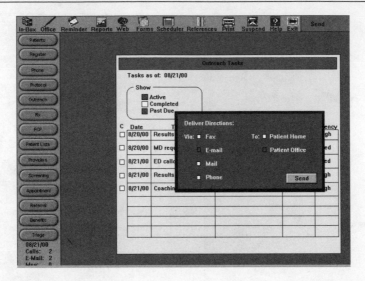

in to see their physician, and the antibiotic therapy is limited to three days. In implementations of the guideline in health care systems that are members of the Institute for Clinical Systems Integration collaborative, treatment success rates are equivalent and costs decreased by as much as 35 percent.[4] First-Rate Health's clinical practice committee reviewed the guideline and decided to adopt all of its elements. They also worked with staff in the access center and clinics to put the guideline into operation as part of telephone triage at the access center.

Adelle calls up the UTI protocol in the system. It guides her through a series of questions that help in determining whether Ms. Richfield is an appropriate patient for the guideline and in ensuring that there are no complicating factors that rule out its use. She records Ms. Richfield's reported symptom of dysuria and that she has no shaking or chills. The system pulls up an encounter note from a follow-up visit for Ms. Richfield's last episode of UTI, which was treated successfully with antibiotic therapy.

Suzanne Richfield has been a managed care patient of First-Rate Health for five years and receives her care there consistently. As part of her orientation, Ms. Richfield completed a detailed health history and health needs assessment that is part of her electronic health record in the Enterprise System. Because First-Rate Health has such a complete patient clinical history in its patient care system, the rules-based decision support in the system is able to scan this information for contraindications such as diabetes, recent hospitalization, or failure of therapy.

FIGURE 5.10. ENTERPRISE SYSTEM VIEWED BY TRIAGE NURSE: UTI TREATMENT PROTOCOL PATIENT RESPONSE SCREEN.

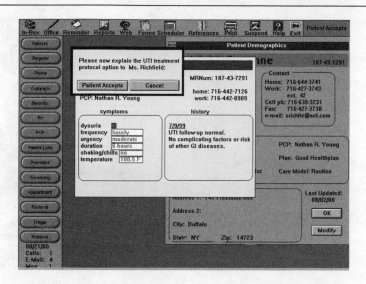

Adelle explains the UTI treatment protocol option to Ms. Richfield, as shown in Figure 5.10, and after hearing that she qualifies for the guideline, Ms. Richfield prefers the option of going directly to the pharmacy to pick up a prescription rather than coming in to see a doctor. Adelle tells her what to do if her symptoms do not subside and offers to send written instructions as well.

Because Ms. Richfield has been on sulfa before without any adverse effects, Adelle activates the standing order established by First-Rate Health's clinical practice committee. After she electronically signs the prescription, the system transmits it to the community pharmacy where Ms. Richfield picks up her medications. Ms. Richfield requests that the patient instructions be faxed to her home. Adelle sets a reminder for herself to call Ms. Richfield in two days to see how she is doing.

Primary Care Physician

Dr. Subeeka Reedy is a PCP in one of First-Rate Health's practice sites. She has seen many improvements in patient management and workflow since the access center was implemented. As she reviews communications in her electronic in-box, the benefits she receives will be illustrated.

The first message concerns one of her patients, who called in requesting an appointment. When the service representative could not find an available appointment

FIGURE 5.11. ENTERPRISE SYSTEM VIEWED BY PRIMARY CARE PHYSICIAN: ACCESS CENTER COMMUNICATION SCREEN.

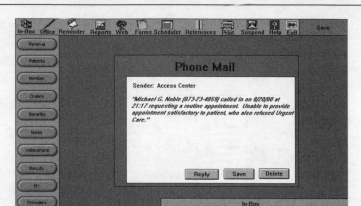

that was soon enough to please the patient, he declined other options, such as an appointment in urgent care. As shown in Figure 5.11, First-Rate Health routinely notifies PCPs of instances such as this so they can determine appropriate follow-up. Subeeka would like to check in on this patient to see what prompted the call. She sets a reminder for herself to call the patient later in the day when she has some administrative time built into her schedule.

Subeeka's second patient, John Adams, called the access center to request a renewal of his prescription for dilantin. Jean Mercer at the access center transcribed and forwarded the message. Subeeka checks the patient summary for Mr. Adams and notes that dilantin levels were last checked more than three months ago. She orders a one-month prescription renewal sent to the community pharmacy where the patient picks up his medications. This pharmacy is not yet electronically connected, so Subeeka authorizes transmission by fax. As shown in Figure 5.12, she also sends a message to the clinic nurse to call the patient, explain that a thirty-day supply of dilantin will be available at the pharmacy, and make arrangements for the laboratory test.

A third message in Subeeka's in-box came in over the Internet from one of her patients, Brian McGraw, who has seen reports in the local newspaper concerning a new treatment for asthma and would like more information. Subeeka has been following these developments through bulletins from First-Rate Health's clinical practice committee and discussions at staff meetings. She searches out a

FIGURE 5.12. ENTERPRISE SYSTEM VIEWED BY PRIMARY CARE PHYSICIAN: REMINDER TO CLINIC NURSE SCREEN.

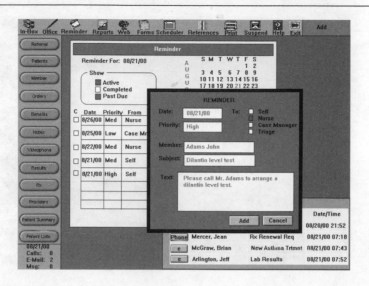

Web site on asthma that is a good source of information on new treatments and adds it to her list of favorites. She then sends a return message to Mr. McGraw advising him that the treatment is still in initial trials but appears promising. She attaches to the message a hot link for the asthma information Web site, as shown in Figure 5.13, so that Mr. McGraw can easily access it.

Patient

Patients of First-Rate Health have gained much easier access to services and information at the Web sites maintained by the health care system. We join Dr. Reedy's patient Brian McGraw at his home PC.

Brian is a member of Good Health Plan, the managed care plan operated by First-Rate Health. He first accesses Good Health Plan's home page and enters his ID and password. (Good Health Plan provides some public information but reserves interactive functions for its members and uses this sign-on procedure to restrict access.) Brian retrieves his message from Dr. Reedy and decides to check out the asthma information Web site immediately. He clicks on the hot link and is connected within a few seconds. After reviewing the services available, shown in Figure 5.14, he decides to subscribe for automatic notification of new information about asthma treatments and other developments. He enrolls in this service,

FIGURE 5.13. ENTERPRISE SYSTEM VIEWED BY PRIMARY CARE PHYSICIAN: REPLY TO PATIENT SCREEN.

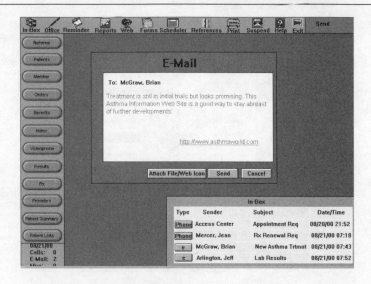

FIGURE 5.14. ENTERPRISE SYSTEM VIEWED BY PATIENT: INTERNET INFORMATION "PUSH" SCREEN.

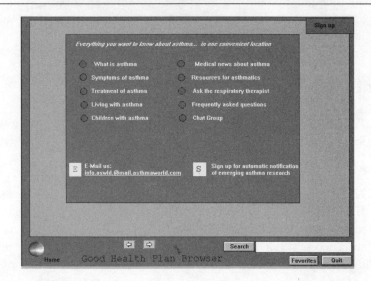

FIGURE 5.15. ENTERPRISE SYSTEM VIEWED BY PATIENT: PRIMARY CARE PHYSICIAN SEARCH SCREEN.

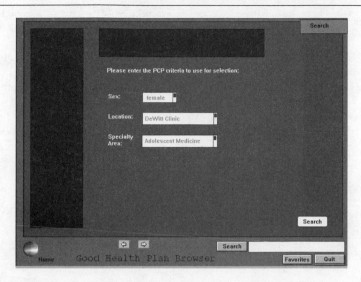

which will now send bulletins to his Internet e-mail address when information about new asthma treatments is published in clinical journals or presented at professional meetings. This will be a convenient way for him to stay informed.

Brian has other business to accomplish today. His daughter wishes to change her PCP, so he clicks on this option on the Good Health Plan Web site. He calls his daughter to join him in the study so that she can make the selection herself. His daughter requests a female physician at the DeWitt Clinic who specializes in adolescent medicine, as shown in Figure 5.15. The system responds with a photograph and some information concerning one of the physicians at that location who has the requested qualifications and whose patient panel is open (she is accepting patients). His daughter accepts Dr. Sorbello as her new PCP, and the information is transmitted to update the managed care member database and to the practice administrator in Dr. Sorbello's office, who will prepare a welcome letter for Dr. Sorbello to sign.

Brian McGraw's teenage son plays soccer and will require physical therapy to strengthen his knee following an injury in the game last week. Brian recalls that there are some special coverage rules regarding physical therapy in his health plan benefits. He clicks on the Benefits button on the Web site and easily locates PT benefits with the aid of an electronic index. He prints a copy of this information so he can refer to it later.

Notes

1. Solberg, L. I., Mosser, G., and McDonald, S. "The Three Faces of Performance Measurement: Improvement, Accountability, and Research." *The Joint Commission Journal on Quality Improvement*, 1997, *23*, 135–147.
2. Mosser, G. "Clinical Process Improvement: Engage First, Measure Later." *Quality Management in Health Care*, 1996, *4*, 11–20.
3. Mosser, G., and Sakowski, J. *1996 Health Care Guidelines*. Vol. 1. Bloomington, Minn.: Institute for Clinical Systems Integration, 1996.
4. O'Connor, P. J., and others. "Mechanism of Action and Impact of a Cystitis Clinical Practice Guideline on Outcomes and Costs of Care in an HMO." *The Joint Commission Journal on Quality Improvement*, 1996, *22*, 673–682.

CHAPTER SIX

CROSS-CONTINUUM CARE MANAGEMENT: NEW MODELS

Jane Metzger

Health care has traditionally been delivered as a series of outpatient encounters and inpatient episodes of care, involving many different individual providers, departments, and settings. Often the patient (and in rare cases the medical record) is the only common thread because care is fragmented across multiple providers and locations. Creating an integrated care process to replace the old process is at the core of the transformation occurring in our health care system. When applied to care delivery, integration requires seamless coordination and continuity along two intersecting axes: the traditional boundaries of health care settings, and traditional functions and disciplines. Thus, conceiving the new process requires starting over from scratch.

In response to (or in anticipation of) providing at-risk care, every health care organization in the United States is in some stage of the substantial rethinking, reorganizing, and retooling required to deliver care in a more integrated way. New models are emerging as integrating health networks deliver at-risk care for large numbers of patients. This is where large numbers of both providers and patients are first gaining actual experience with integrated, cross-continuum care.

The initial focus of care management is on high-risk patients (usually defined as those with one or more chronic diseases). This is the logical starting point because these are the patients who are least well-served by our traditional, fragmented process. As a result, patients with chronic conditions substantially dominate the utilization of health care resources (and costs of care), as illustrated in the following estimates:[1]

Service	*Percentage of Utilization by Patients Who Are High-Risk*
Home care visits	96.1
Prescriptions	83.3
Hospital days	79.9
Visits to other professionals	70.3
Hospital admissions	68.6
Physician visits	66.0
Emergency department visits	55.1

Any health care organization with the ability to examine population-based utilization for single or multiple settings recognizes a similar pattern: A relatively small number of patients utilizes the most services.[2, 3] This utilization places any health care system at significant financial risk once it provides at-risk care.

The extent of activity to develop and implement new models for care management is reflected in the recent published literature, which shares ideas and lessons learned. In addition, several national coalitions of health care organizations are working jointly to share knowledge and accelerate progress. There are, however, no compilations of experience from which one can glean a picture of the complete process: the activities, the players, and the organizational challenges.

This chapter is an attempt to create such a description based on the analysis of case examples of implemented models. Sources of information included the following:

- Prior research conducted by First Consulting Group's Emerging Practices Group
- Review of the literature
- Visits and interviews with staff responsible for new models of integrated high-risk patient management in several of our collaborator organizations
- Case examples from client engagements that involve information technology planning, implementation, or operational effectiveness of new care delivery models
- Visits or telephone consultations with staff at identified organizations that operate highly integrated models
- Conferences and publications of two national coalitions, the National Chronic Care Consortium and the Chronic Care in HMOs Initiative

This discussion focuses on emerging models for high-risk patients because this is clearly the population being initially targeted. As we note, emerging models differ in terms of the aspects of care they encompass and the extent to which new elements are integrated into the process of care. Our research focused on understanding the highly integrated model based in primary care because this is the model being created in the integrated health care systems that have the most experience with managed care. (Not surprisingly we found virtually all implemented models in HMOs, IDNs that operate a health plan, and IDNs that have gained experience in providing Medicare managed care.) We believe that the model of these early adopters will diffuse to all IDNs.

A few organizations have begun to extend the new models beyond high-risk patients. In doing so, they have utilized a subset of the process activities of the models for high-risk patients or apply activities less intensively, rather than using a totally different set of activities and process. This suggests that once we understand and put into operation highly integrated models for high-risk patients, we will have learned much of what we need to know about the process to more broadly extend the principles of cross-continuum management.

Definitions

Terminology concerning new models for management of high-risk patients is currently not used consistently. Exhibit 6.1 provides definitions for the terms used in this chapter. These terms are generally consistent with the terminology employed in the identified national collaborations working on chronic disease management. Our topic, care management, overlaps with *disease management* when the definition for the latter includes both a new process for patient management and new clinical content (such as patient education materials or protocols to guide patient management). Care management is also the same as the high-end definition of medical management, as described in Exhibit 6.1, which can include ongoing case management integrated into the care process.

Care Management Principles of New Models

Exhibit 6.2 summarizes the principles underlying new models for cross-continuum management of high-risk patients. The core principle is population-based management. The premise is simply that different populations of patients have different medical and psychosocial needs that must be addressed in order to achieve good outcomes.[4, 5] Patient populations are subdivided into clinically relevant subgroups; they may be defined according to a common medical condition such as diabetes or chronic pulmonary disease, on the basis of decreased capability for self-management and at risk for declining functional status (for example, frail elderly), or according to patterns of obtaining health services (for example, medically underserved populations such as Medicaid patients). Providing population-based care manage-

EXHIBIT 6.1. OVERLAPPING DEFINITIONS OF NEW MODELS.

Cross-continuum care management: Systematic approach to providing a supportive network of coordinated services and resources tailored to meet the medical needs and interests of each member/patient. More intensive management is involved for members/patients with chronic conditions that require ongoing management (e.g., asthma, diabetes, chronic obstructive pulmonary disease, congestive heart failure); or with personal, health behavior, or environmental characteristics that indicate they are at risk of decreasing functional status or high-cost care (e.g., frail elderly). More intensive care management typically includes primary care case management. (See below.)

Disease management: A systematic approach to managing members/patients who have specific chronic medical conditions with the goal of producing the best outcomes in the most cost-effective manner. Disease management typically addresses education and other support for patients with chronic conditions who manage their own health reliably and targets additional interventions, based on disease-specific protocols, for patients at "high risk" or complications or decreased functional status. (Most programs described as "disease management" include only individual components such as patient education or care protocols, rather than a comprehensive care model.)

Primary care case management: Provider role responsible for assessing patient status, environment, and self-management capacity and then planning, organizing, implementing, and coordinating assistance and health care services to respond to the needs of patients with complex medical and psychosocial needs. This role involves extensive education/coaching of patients and family members to empower them in personal health management as well as intensive follow-up to monitor completion of care management interventions and patient status and progress. Typically, a nurse case manager works closely with the patient's primary care physician or clinical team, taking responsibility for assisting the patient and monitoring progress on an ongoing basis.

Medical management: Process implemented by health care organizations and health plans to monitor and manage the utilization of health care resources of participating (contract) health care providers. Traditionally, the focus of medical management has been on reducing the costs of care; typical functions include utilization review (pre-admit, admit authorization, LOS assignment), case management during hospitalization, and referral management. Emerging approaches guide the care process more actively through clinical protocols/pathways, care standards, decision support, and high-risk case management. Generally, health plans develop and enforce medical management policies and procedures. However, large medical groups and IDNs increasingly seek to develop and enforce their own programs in exchange for a larger capitated rate from the health plans with whom they contract.

EXHIBIT 6.2. BASIC PRINCIPLES OF INTEGRATED PRIMARY CARE MANAGEMENT OF HIGH-RISK PATIENTS.

Population-based Management	• Populations of patients characterized as subgroups with distinct medical and psychosocial characteristics

Care Models	• Care models adapted to meet the needs of subgroups of patients
	  – How care is accessed and delivered
	  – What care is delivered

Protocols	• Guidelines/protocols based on demonstrated epidemiologic evidence
Team Work	• Care management that emphasizes the coordinated interplay of a set of competencies and integrates primary and specialty care in a unified process
Primary Care Case Management	• Assistance to patients in meeting health management goals from a case manager who arranges and coordinates care and follows patient progress closely
Cross-continuum	• All services coordinated and provided in the least intensive setting, including home- and community-based services
Personal Health Management	• Patients guided/coached to adopt best practices in personal health management

ment requires first stratifying the population into meaningful subgroups based on their needs. Then the health care system sets up a patient management structure and process—a care model with the appropriate access, resources, and expertise to address the needs of the identified subgroups of patients.[2, 3, 6–10]

Another key component is evidence-based care protocols, which offer a starting point for developing an individualized care plan for each patient.[4, 5, 9, 11] These protocols provide recommended methods and content for assessments, treatments, and services shown to achieve improvements in the targeted population. When care management protocols are implemented consistently, including documentation of variances and outcomes, they can be improved on an ongoing basis as more experience is gained. The goal for most health care systems, to derive their own experience-based protocols, awaits further advances in data capture and population-based outcomes analysis before it can be realized.

Effective management of high-risk (often chronic care) patients requires the coordination and interplay of many competencies. Therefore, another principle underlying new care models is integration of primary and specialty care. In many models, this involves a primary care physician (PCP) in the lead role, with one or more specialists, as necessary, participating in patient assessment and care planning. The rationale for this structure is that patient management ideally reflects both the generalist approach to managing the complex interplay of medical and social factors and the expert management of the medical conditions. In other models, a specialist physician (such as a pulmonologist, endocrinologist, or cardiologist) serves as the patient's PCP. In addition, nurse case managers, social workers, and respiratory and other therapists all have competencies that should be integrated, with the result that the care team is multidisciplinary and teamwork is key.[12]

Primary care case management provides high-risk patients with support and assistance in arranging care and services in all settings and with close follow-up. The objective is to ensure that progress goals are met whenever possible and that the patient's care team can intervene quickly when the care plan should be modified. This assistance is over and above what can reasonably be achieved for high-risk patients by a PCP in the more traditional model for managed care.

Coordinated, proactive approaches to ongoing management that use case managers to follow patients closely are not totally new. Behavioral health has been employing case management to ensure continuity of care and to minimize needs for intensive intervention for a decade or more;[13, 14, 15] public and community health models have employed active outreach, tracking, and follow-up for at-risk populations or patients with communicable diseases since before World War I and continue to do so today[16]; and public and private programs for AIDS patients have employed case management to enhance quality of life and health outcomes for that patient population.[17, 18, 19] Today the case manager role and many of the same principles are being extended and integrated into routine care for patients with chronic disease.

The goal of care for the chronically ill is generally to halt or reverse a progression toward increasing functional limitation. This leads in most cases to a focus on functional status and quality of life rather than to a cure. The care team tracks functional status as a major measure of status and progress, seeks to reflect patient preferences, and places a priority on delivering care in the most convenient setting. Doing so requires integrating medical services with home- and community-based services.[12]

Finally, active participation and empowerment of patients and family members through education and coaching makes them more effective at personal health management and achieving maximum possible independence and quality of life.[12]

Organizational Models

Highly integrated models for high-risk patient management are organized within the care system in three different ways:

• Through integration into primary care practices, with the PCP assisted by a primary care case manager and a care team that may include one or more specialist physicians and other providers such as respiratory therapists and social workers.[20, 21, 22, 23, 24] Regular team meetings to discuss patients enrolled in intensive care management and coordinated appointments for these patients to see multiple team members during an encounter are common.

• In separate ambulatory practices or clinics focused on patient populations defined by chronic disease or age.[6, 25, 26, 27] These are staffed with multiple specialist or PCPs, primary care case managers, and other care team members, as discussed earlier. Some of these models include advanced practice nurses who assume more patient clinical management duties for patients enrolled in intensive care management. Special sites of this type are often established to support Medicare managed care.

• As miniclinics or group clinics organized within a primary care site.[5, 28–32] In this model, certain times during the week are set aside for high-risk patients. Patients meet with their clinical teams, which assemble at the primary care site, or as a support group that includes all of their clinical team members. Patients who participate in group clinics also have individual discussions or appointments with one or more members of their clinical teams.

The processes for care management of high-risk patients are similar in all of these organizational models, with the exception that in the third model, routine patient encounters with the health care system include some group sessions.

Typical Processes

Figure 6.1 presents a schematic of the highly integrated models for managing high-risk patients that organizes the process into four phases. Figure 6.2 lists the key activities in each phase in more detail. The first phase is quite different from traditional models for care delivery, but in the subsequent phases many of the steps appear similar. For high-risk patients assigned to primary care case management, however, there are major differences in the allocation of responsibilities among members of an extended care team and the intensity and frequency of interactions with care providers.

Case Finding and Intake

The ideal time to identify patients for high-risk care management is the first time they come to the attention of the care system—when they enroll. Other

FIGURE 6.1. OVERVIEW OF THE PROCESS FOR CROSS-CONTINUUM MANAGEMENT OF HIGH-RISK PATIENTS.

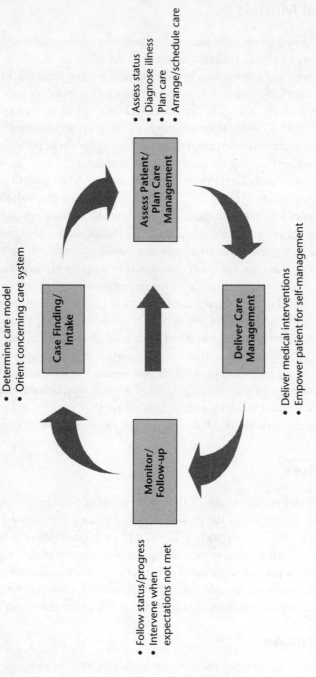

Case Finding/Intake
- Identify risk profile
- Bring patients into contact
- Determine care model
- Orient concerning care system

Assess Patient/Plan Care Management
- Assess status
- Diagnose illness
- Plan care
- Arrange/schedule care

Deliver Care Management
- Deliver medical interventions
- Empower patient for self-management

Monitor/Follow-up
- Follow status/progress
- Intervene when expectations not met

FIGURE 6.2. OVERVIEW OF THE PROCESS PHASES AND ACTIVITIES FOR CROSS-CONTINUUM MANAGEMENT OF HIGH-RISK PATIENTS.

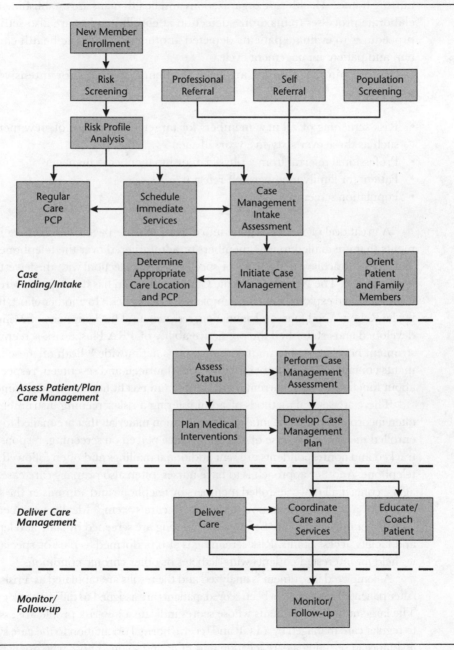

opportunities, in decreasing order of preference, are the following: first encounter with a PCP, first encounter with specialist physician, long-term care, hospital, and nursing home.[33] Health care organizations and health plans are establishing rather elaborate processes to maximize detection at enrollment but are also setting up procedures to evaluate patients detected at other points in the health care system and patient management cycle.

Four main mechanisms are used to identify patients for intensive care management:

- Risk screening of all new members (or targeted subgroups of new members such as those over sixty-five years of age)
- Professional referral from a physician or inpatient case manager
- Patient (or family member) self-referral
- Population screening

A great deal of work has gone into developing one-page risk-screening instruments that are mailed to new members or administered over the telephone.[33, 34, 35] The goal is to achieve a high level of specificity (risk detection) with the fewest questions possible. The National Chronic Care Consortium has developed a screening instrument and explored numerous implementation issues.[33] In another effort, funded by the Robert Wood Johnson Foundation, researchers at the University of Minnesota developed and established the predictive ability of PRA Plus, a risk-screening instrument now licensed to many organizations nationwide.[35] Both of these instruments contain a small number of questions (fourteen and seventeen, respectively) about functional status, current medications, and recent health care encounters.

There are several methods of administering a risk-screening instrument. It is often incorporated into the intake and orientation materials that are mailed to newly enrolled members. Because of the importance placed on screening, responses are tracked and nonrespondents are sent additional mailings and often followed up by telephone. Another approach is to have nurses (often also primary care case managers) contact all newly enrolled members by telephone and administer the survey as part of a general orientation to the health care system.[36] Ideally, new members who call or appear for care before risk screening are screened by staff at telephone and facility access points. Risk screening is also performed as part of special clinics held for interested patients with diabetes or other chronic conditions.[30]

A completed instrument is analyzed and the results are tabulated as a risk score. After patient responses have been scored, patients are assigned to different risk groups. The large number of patients whose scores indicate a low-risk profile are assigned to regular care managed by a PCP and receive normal orientation to the care system, assistance in selecting a care location and PCP, and so on. Those who appear to require immediate medical attention or who are candidates for primary care case management are contacted (in person at the patient's home or by telephone) to obtain additional information about their environment, recent medical history, and so on. Immediate medical care is arranged and case management initiated as appropriate.

Nurse case managers usually manage the risk-screening process (and in some models administer the screening questions by telephone to some or all patients). They usually are involved in scoring and following up with patients whose initial risk profiles require further evaluation. At one health care system, each primary care site has an access nurse whose job is to contact all new members, perform risk screening, and assist with PCP selection and enrollment in case management, when appropriate.[20]

Risk screening is used to sort patients into several different categories: the healthy, the worried well, those with chronic disease that is being managed, those with chronic disease that is not being managed well (the symptoms are not being managed), and those at truly high risk of deteriorating function (seriously impaired, constantly changing disease and treatment). Most organizations are initially focusing more intensive care management on patients who are stratified into the last two groups.[37]

Professional referrals can come from physicians in any setting and often from inpatient nurse case managers who discharge patients. In a survey of twenty HMOs with Medicare risk contracts, all identified the majority of care management patients via referrals.[38] In one health care system, any managed care patient admitted to a hospital with congestive heart failure is evaluated by a case manager in the cross-continuum disease management program.[25] Other modes of entry in some organizations are one-day screening clinics provided at no charge to the patient,[30] or an order for home care.

Health care organizations and health plans generally have rather specific criteria for patient eligibility for intensive care management. For example, one health care system includes patients with any of the following criteria in its high-risk management program:[20]

- Recent need for acute care (admitted to hospital, skilled nursing facility, or rehab within the past six months and greater than seventy years of age or unplanned readmission within the last thirty days)

- Disease burden or functional disability (four or more chronic diagnoses, two or more emergency room visits within twelve months, chronic use of more than four medications, impaired performance of activities of daily living and no support for addressing needs, or frail elder at risk)

- Other diagnoses (such as Alzheimer's disease or dementia, cancer, or traumatic brain injury)

Staff involved in managing these programs report that once physicians see the benefits to their patients, they refer those who do not meet all of the criteria because they believe that a broader population could benefit from closer coordination and monitoring.[21] Patients and family members can also self-refer, and organizations use newsletters and other forms of community education to acquaint the patient population with the availability and purpose of these programs.

When information systems permit, organizations also identify candidate patients by screening service utilization information to detect patients with underlying medical conditions that could benefit from closer management. Some conditions can be detected from laboratory results (for example, newly diagnosed diabetes). Given the immaturity or local nature of clinical systems, claims data (or "dummy" claims/encounter data) are often used for broader screening. HCFA 1500 and UB82/92 forms include diagnoses and procedures, as well as dates of service for an episode of care. Examples of screening criteria are more than one chronic condition, more than two emergency room encounters, more than four outpatient encounters, more than one admission in the past year; or a specified number of prescriptions. Obviously the broader the coverage of enterprise services in the billing or claims database, the better will be the population screening according to these types of criteria.

Six of twenty surveyed HMOs with Medicare risk contracts reported using their corporate computer databases to identify appropriate enrollees. One site uses a nightly scan of ICD-9 codes recorded at office visits during the previous day to flag patients for further review by a case management supervisor.[38]

As part of a program for early detection of patients with Type II diabetes, one health care system is using an educational video describing the risk factors and encouraging members to contact a health promotion center for additional information and to enroll in a counseling program.[30] In the future, opportunities for risk screening and general information are likely to be offered via kiosks in public areas of health care organizations, employer sites, and public access sites in libraries and shopping centers. In addition, as Internet technology and Web sites become more integrated into routine communication between patients and their insurance and health care providers, these vehicles will provide additional ways for patients to assess their health risk factors and report pertinent information to their care providers. (Patient communication options are discussed further in Chapter Seven.)

Referral history is another approach to screening. One IDN queries claims to identify patients in the top 10 percent in terms of costs of care, with more than $2,000 for outpatient care or more than $10,000 in total care per year. The system produces a printout listing the referral history, which gives a good overview of what is happening with each identified patient. Case managers at the site where the patient routinely receives care review this information, consult medical records, and contact PCPs and patients for further evaluation.[20]

Assess Patient Status and Plan Care Management

For patients enrolled in intensive care management, the case manager often begins a detailed case management assessment before the first encounter with the physician (it may even occur during a home visit or telephone conversation as part of risk screening/intake). This initial assessment generally includes the patient's understanding and perception of his or her disease and status, the patient's ability to manage self-care and engage in activities of daily living, social support environment, and so on.

Problem behaviors identified in the assessment are addressed by interventions to encourage and support the patient in altering behavior. For example, a diabetic patient who is not complying with prescribed insulin might be targeted for different types of education (including group education), with the goal that the patient will take insulin as prescribed to manage his or her illness. Behavioral areas addressed include health access, safety, medications, treatments, and outcomes. For each area, goal-oriented case management interventions are intended to reduce barriers and enhance success. The case manager incorporates these interventions into a case management plan for the patient. (Chapter Eight features an example of a care model that leverages system-supported protocols to develop a case management plan.)

Planning medical care for patients in care management programs is typically interdisciplinary. At a minimum, it involves the PCP and case manager, often one or more specialist physicians, and possibly a social worker. Some organizations are starting to include clinical pharmacists as regular team members or on a consultant basis because many patients in these programs take numerous medications. Typically, regular team meetings are scheduled each week. In one evaluation of the Program of All-Inclusive Care of the Elderly, staff devoted eight hours each week to formal multidisciplinary meetings to assess patient progress and discuss management options for their patients.[39]

Patients and family members are ideally full collaborators in selecting medical management options and in developing the care and case management plans. Adapting plans to patient and family member preferences increases compliance and successful outcomes.[40] Some programs also include patient contracts regarding self-management activities and goals.

The structure of care management plans is typically time-based and includes frequent scheduled reassessments through testing and ambulatory encounters with the care team. (A major role of the primary care case manager is to ensure that all services are scheduled and all medications and other treatments are obtained.)

Programs targeting chronic disease almost always employ problem- or condition-based protocols that lay out both recommended medical interventions and the desired frequency of reassessment and follow-up. Because most of these patients have multiple chronic problems to be managed and many specific patient characteristics to take into account, substantial combining and customizing of care protocols is often required to develop a plan of care for each patient. This makes protocols formatted as pathways less applicable for acute care than for procedures such as hip replacements, for which care can be more standardized.[41] Having a written plan detailing interventions and expectations regarding progress (rather than merely orders for interventions) is important for continuity of care and for monitoring status and outcomes.[42] Plans of care based on protocols can also be vehicles for automatic preauthorization of services when prenegotiated with a health plan.[43]

Some care management protocols are structured in the format of clinical pathways.[43] In some, algorithms and branching logic specify changes in medical and patient self-management when desired outcomes are not achieved. An example is a comprehensive diabetes management program[26] in which thirty-two protocols cover management and tracking of patients treated with diet, sulfonylurea agents, and/or insulin. Protocols also guide treatment of lipid disorders, gestational diabetes, impaired glucose tolerance, diabetes in pregnancy, and complications such as hypertension and nephropathy. Nurse practitioners (guided by a diabetologist) see patients quarterly and with the diabetologist at least once a year. Patients are referred to a dietitian upon entry and to ophthalmology on a recurring basis. Based on the findings (laboratory results or other measurements or observations) in each encounter, the protocols lay out changes in the care plan from that point forward.

The National Chronic Care Consortium has developed the Extended Care Pathway (ECP) to provide a framework for "a standardized approach to the multidisciplinary care of an individual with a particular diagnosis."[44] The ECP is a care-planning and management mechanism that covers all settings over an extended period of time and integrates care by identifying the responsibilities of all members of the extended care team. For different stages of health status (asymptomatic, symptomatic, functional decline, functional recovery, adjustment), the ECP defines assessments, interventions, goals, outcomes to be measured, and information to be transferred. Ideally the ECP spans settings of care (including the patient's home) and provides for a smooth and coordinated transition for both the care team and the patient. The ECP differs from clinical pathways, which are primarily implemented for procedure-based inpatient care, in that it incorporates the full range of psychosocial assessments, goals, and interventions (some of which are otherwise recorded in the case management plan); it spans settings of care and incorporates roles of community-based care providers, as appropriate; and for continuity of care, it defines content and methods of sharing information among sites when patients are transferred.

Deliver Care Management

The major difference in care delivery for patients who are enrolled in a high-risk management program is the involvement of the primary care case manager. This role coordinates and arranges services and devotes extra attention to ensuring that barriers to compliance (for example, lack of transportation and poor understanding) are identified and addressed.

The Case Management Society of America, which has developed standards of practice for case management, includes "facilitator" and "advocate" as two important aspects of the role.[40] In functioning as a facilitator, a case manager actively promotes communication and collaboration among the patient, family, and members of the patient's extended care team; the goal in care coordination is to streamline the care process, focusing on "the best treatment or approach for the client."[40] In functioning as an advocate, the case manager attempts to meet the client's individualized needs and to "represent the client's best interests."[40] Care settings include the home, and many case managers visit patients regularly, in addition to visiting nurses, home health aides, and other providers.

Case management interventions are frequent and numerous, with case managers spending as much as half of their time in face-to-face contact with their patients.[6] Interventions in a patient's case management plan can address practical issues such as arranging transportation to a care site, providing safety assessment of the home, setting up home visits to provide education, monitoring compliance with medications, arranging care in many settings, and coordinating community-based services. Financial issues such as exploring community-based assistance programs and obtaining authorizations can be addressed as well.[6]

Education programs—to increase awareness and knowledge of the disease as well as to empower patients in effective self-management—are a core element. Patient education is typically provided in group and individual settings at physicians' practices, clinics, and community sites as well as at home. Case managers often provide much of the patient education and coaching, and use frequent telephone conversations to reinforce the importance of personal and health care system interventions and compliance. Some models use education specialists in the particular disease. An increasing number of support groups and electronic chat groups are being established or facilitated by health care organizations as an adjunct to direct care services.[7, 30] Group clinic sessions included in some models provide an opportunity for both patient education and peer support.[31]

Case managers arrange for services, both within the IDN and from community and other service providers. In one survey of Medicare HMO providers with case management,[45] case managers engaged in the following activities:

Arranging HMO services   100 percent

Educating enrollee   91 percent

Advising/counseling family   74 percent

Helping with health decisions   70 percent

Arranging self-pay services   70 percent

Arranging other-pay services   65 percent

Making home visits   61 percent

Case managers document every interaction with patients, family members, providers, and provider organizations. In some programs (57 percent in the survey just mentioned), they contribute their plans and notes to patients' medical records. Case managers typically provide periodic written communication for patient PCPs, even if they maintain separate case management records.

Monitor Patients and Follow-Up

The primary care case manager assumes the major responsibility for following patients on an ongoing basis. The frequency of regular contact is usually specified by the case management protocol and includes encounters in the clinic or practice, home visits, and telephone follow-up.

As part of monitoring, case managers attempt to confirm that planned interventions such as treatments occur, and to identify and follow up unplanned events such as visits to the emergency room or urgent care clinic. Improving compliance with medications, treatments, and self-management interventions is a major factor in improving patient outcomes. One estimate pegs medication noncompliance rates as high as 43 percent for the general population and 55 percent among the elderly.[46] For patients with asthma, noncompliance with recommended treatment may be even greater.[47]

In the absence of information technology assistance, case managers rely heavily on regular conversations with patients and family members to check on medication compliance, as well as to determine whether other aspects of the care management plan are on course. In the survey of twenty HMOs with Medicare risk contracts, 96 percent used telephone calls to track patients, 70 percent used office visits, and 61 percent used home visits.[45]

The primary care case manager is responsible for obtaining updates from community care providers such as visiting nurses (who are often in the most frequent contact with the patient) and for communicating with the patient's PCP or clinical team about patient progress and any changes in status. Case managers expect patients and family members to call when they have questions or need to report changes; patient education materials often include information about indications for calling the care system. Case managers in some programs carry beepers or have scheduled coverage during off hours and weekends. Ideally, patient medical records for patients in intensive care management programs are tagged or patient registration displays in computer systems are flagged so that staff at telephone and facility access points can notify the appropriate case manager when patients call or appear for unscheduled care.

Primary care case managers also follow patients when they are hospitalized or in rehab or skilled nursing facilities after they are discharged. In integrated systems of cross-continuum care (discussed shortly), they work closely with episode case managers in the hospital or rehabilitation center rather than directly coordinating services in these settings themselves. Especially important for close coordination with institutional case managers, of course, is discharge planning, which encompasses all post-discharge care and services, including home care.

Health Care System Staff Roles in Integrated Models for High-Risk Patients

Typical Roles Based in Primary Care

In integrated models for managing high-risk patients, responsibilities for specific tasks are typically shared among the patient's primary physician, a primary care case manager, and an extended care team that includes specialist physicians and other providers. The key roles are summarized in Table 6.1. As in the traditional managed care model, patients receive their care from a designated physician or clinical team. If the physician is a PCP, the clinical team for the patient is likely to include one or more specialists. Specialty physicians can also serve as the designated primary physician (for example, a pulmonologist acting as primary physician for a patient with severe chronic asthma). Another model for physician staffing is a team of roving specialists who provide physician education and see patients jointly with PCPs. Yet another approach has stable patients managed by PCPs and unstable patients by specialists (periodically or on an ongoing basis, as needed).

The primary care case manager is responsible for ongoing management of patients enrolled in intensive care management, including some monitoring and coordination with episode case managers when patients are hospitalized. This role is pivotal to the more proactive management model. In some models, case managers specialize in the care of patients with a particular condition (for example, diabetes or HIV/AIDS); in others, case managers are generalists and manage patients with a range of chronic conditions.[48] Typically, case managers work as team members with a number of primary physicians or clinical teams in managing high-risk patients. They tend to be registered nurses with prior experience in home care, in community medicine, or in working with the target patient population (for example, frail elderly, AIDS patients, children with severe disabilities, or women with high-risk pregnancies). Some models use social workers or clinical dietitians[30] as case managers or as adjunct members of the clinical team.[48]

In some models advanced practice nurses serve as primary care case managers but assume more responsibility for independent clinical management of patients. Advanced practice nurses include nurse practitioners, who are generally certified in geronotology or other relevant clinical disciplines, and clinical nurse specialists (for example, those who have had intensive training in diabetes management and are certified in diabetes education).[25, 26, 49]

In some models, a case or care management assistant assists the case manager by arranging services, dealing with community agencies, and performing other coordination and communication tasks.

TABLE 6.1. TYPICAL STAFF ROLES IN CROSS-CONTINUUM CARE MANAGEMENT OF HIGH-RISK PATIENTS.

ROLE	DESCRIPTION	KEY ACTIVITIES
Primary MD/ Clinical Team (PMD)	• Primary care or specialist • Responsible for clinical management of an identified group of patients • Assisted by PCCM for designated high-risk patients	• Assess/document patient status/progress • Obtain relevant best practices • Diagnose illness • Collaborate with patient in review of alternatives • Develop/document care plan • Ensure plans meet member preferences • Initiate care delivery (order interventions in care plan) • Educate patient
Primary Care Case Manager (PCCM)	• RN (or social worker) • Manages an identified group of patients on an ongoing basis • Collaborates with PMD/ Team in planning care and monitoring patient status/ progress • Responsible for implementing interventions in case management plan • Typically, first point of entry for patient to care system	• Assess screened patients and determine need for high-risk management program • Perform intake of eligible patients into program • Assess/document patient status/progress • Obtain relevant best practices • Perform case management assessment • Develop case management plan • Arrange/schedule care • Authorize services for coverage and payment • Provide relevant information to patient • Coach patient regarding care plan/follow-up • Monitor completion of services • Monitor member compliance • Deliver/document care • Perform/document case management interventions • Communicate with care team • Discharge from case management
Advanced Practice Nurse PCCM	• All of the above • Takes on more direct clinical responsibility	• All of the above • Develop/document careplan • Initiate care delivery
Case/Care Management Assistant	• Assists with arrangements for care and case management interventions	• Arrange care/services • Follow up with patient • Document interactions

Other Roles in Ambulatory Care

Several other role definitions for case management were identified in our research. Generally these roles focus a dedicated nurse or other staff person on a subset of the activities normally performed by a primary care case manager, as described earlier. They occur in models in which either a broad range of functions is subdivided into separate roles (as opposed to being performed by a single individual) or the patient management model includes only a subset of activities such as patient education or care coordination.

Another role, mentioned previously, is the access nurse. Assigned to each clinic or practice site, the access nurse contacts new members who have selected the clinic or practice or a local PCP, provides orientation to the procedures of the health care system, and performs initial screening to identify patients in need of health care services or who are possible candidates for case management. New enrollees who have not selected a PCP are assisted in choosing one by the access nurse, who also contacts inactive patients.[20]

Another role is the telemanagement nurse. In one program, telemanagement nurses are assigned to a special clinic that has been established to assist recently discharged congestive heart failure patients via telephone. The call frequency is set according to a standard protocol, starting at several times a week and decreasing if the patient appears to be stable or improving. Nurses assess patient status during the conversations and reinforce teaching on self-management. When a nurse discovers a patient who is deteriorating or not making sufficient progress, the patient is sent to a special heart failure clinic for an intensive workup and follow-up.[50] Other telemanagement roles are focused on medication compliance and coaching in self-management.[51]

Patient education and coaching are key activities in chronic disease management programs. One model utilizes nurse patient educators with specialized expertise in a particular chronic disease who travel among practice sites to provide education in conjunction with patient clinic visits.[7]

Another role, the care coordinator, performs only the coordination functions of a primary care case manager, mainly assisting patients in arranging home-based care. This person coordinates among HMO departments, providers of purchased services, and community resources with the goal of providing a seamless system of care resources and community services for the patient. Care coordinators have a nursing, social work, or related degree and typically have experience in home- or community-based care.

The care coordinator is an important role in Social HMOs that integrate acute and chronic care, expanding Medicare coverage to include community-based long-term care.[52] This role is also found in IPA programs, where the IPA holds a Medicare risk contract and hires case managers to assist patients managed by physicians in affiliated physician practices whose care is covered under the risk contract.[53] In this model, the case manager is less likely to work in the physician practice site and is not involved in other aspects of arranging or coordinating care. This makes it more difficult for the physician and case manager to communicate about patients in the program and for the two to establish a close working relationship. Another challenge presented by this model is that only patients with a particular insurance coverage are eligible for case-management assistance.

In some models, a care coordinator assistant makes arrangements for needed services.[54] Because these tasks are so time-consuming, care coordinator assistants enable case managers to handle larger case loads.

The role of volunteer is becoming important in some sites with high-risk management programs. Volunteers supplement staff resources in care models for the frail elderly (by providing in-home assistance and routine communication), for AIDS patients, and for Medicaid programs (in new outreach models). One health care system uses volunteers in a variety of capacities to assist homebound members, to call or send greetings to members, and to participate in health fairs and at the service center.[32] Some models for Medicaid patients use health advocates to perform new-member orientation and follow-up, including frequent home visits if patients are not easily reached by telephone.[8]

Other Roles in Integrated Systems of Cross-Continuum Care

Highly evolved integrated systems of care management provide an overall structure across all sites and settings of care, as shown in Figure 6.3. For every managed care patient, one physician team or clinical team is designated (or selected by the patient) to assume overall responsibility for managing the patient's health. For each high-risk patient, the primary care case manager who assists the PCP is also designated to provide case management on an ongoing basis. As the figure shows, the system of care includes inpatient care settings, rehabilitation, and custodial care, each of which is covered by episode case managers. The episode case manager follows the patient through an episode of institutional care in the acute care or transitional setting such as a skilled nursing or rehabilitation facility. Traditionally, episode case management has been a function of medical management (concurrent utilization review), but the role now increasingly combines utilization management and care management. Some organizations also have case managers covering patients who are hospitalized out of area, and catastrophic patients.[6] When routine or high-risk patients require hospitalization or other institutional care, the day-to-day management responsibility is transferred to the episode case managers and medical staff in that setting, who eventually discharge the patient back to the PCP or, for patients in intensive care management, to the PCP and the primary care case manager.

During an institutional care episode of a high-risk patient, the primary care case manager communicates periodically with the episode case manager. Primary care

FIGURE 6.3. INTEGRATED SYSTEM OF CROSS-CONTINUUM CARE MANAGEMENT.

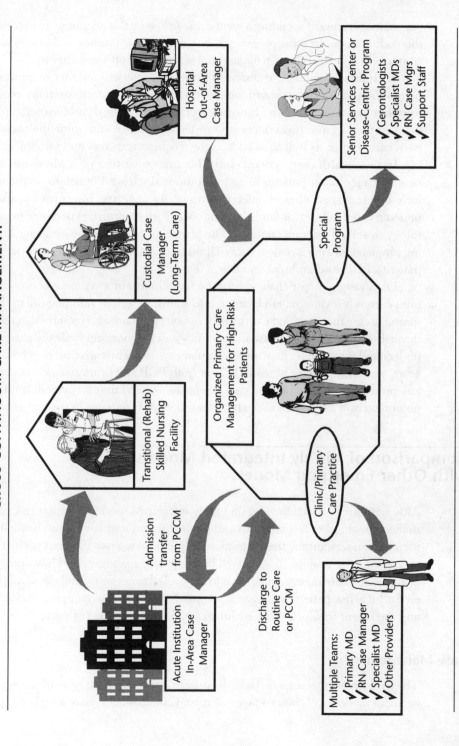

case managers report spending a great deal of time on the telephone to accomplish this coordination. In some programs they carry cellular phones so that they can be contacted while en route to patients' homes and other off-site locations.

Each time a patient is transferred from one facility to another or from inpatient to outpatient status, coordination and handoffs of information are required to ensure continuity of care. Process governance (standards and ownership) and detailed policies and procedures are needed to manage and guide the process in each care setting, as well as to address the frequent transfers and handoffs.

In one health care system, clinical teams consisting of a physician and a case manager follow patients in each institutional setting. Physicians on the teams have different specialties in different settings, for example, internists in subacute or acute care facilities, or family practitioners with extensive experience in gerontology in skilled nursing facilities. The physician becomes the exclusive attending physician during a patient's stay. Upon discharge, responsibility returns to the patient's PCP (and ambulatory clinical team).[6]

Obviously, a major challenge for the participants in a system of cross-continuum care is tracking patient location and status, as well as handing off to the responsible case manager and care team. Continuity of care also requires that the staff throughout the health care system (especially at telephone and facility access points) understand the patient's care model (regular care or an intensive management program) and the manager or team (PCP or both PCP and primary case manager) at any point. One survey of Medicare programs showed that 30 percent used computer flags and 17 percent used chart flags to identify patients in the program.[45]

Comparison of Highly Integrated Models with Other Emerging Models

Although our research focused on highly integrated models for high-risk patient management, other less intensive and less integrated approaches are being implemented. Understanding these variations requires taking two different perspectives: considering the multiple roles played by nurse case managers and how integrated primary care case management fits into the overall framework; and classifying models for high-risk patient management according to the care components included and the extent to which these are integrated into the process of care.

Case Management

The term *case manager* is applied fairly broadly to staff in different types of patient management models and covers a range of roles. Case managers have long been used in the inpatient setting to ensure that patient stays are managed according to the rules of insurance carriers and that all payer-required communications of information on patient diagnosis and status occur at the appropriate times (which is mainly a financial and utilization management function).[41] In terms of integration into the patient clinical management process, this traditional role represents the opposite end of the spectrum from integrated primary care case management. Key characteristics of these two extremes of the spectrum are compared in Table 6.2. Case manager roles can fall at points along the continuum between integrated primary care case management and concurrent utilization management. One way of differentiating a program focused on care management from one focused on utilization management or service coordination is the number of patients per case manager and the amount of time spent in direct patient interaction. In the survey of twenty HMOs with Medicare risk contracts, 14 percent reported that case managers have caseloads of fewer than twenty patients, whereas 17 percent have caseloads in excess of 120 patients.[45] Those with small caseloads interact frequently with patients and spend considerable time each week tracking individual patients. Those with much larger caseloads obviously are able to devote considerably less time and attention to each patient. Organizations with an integrated system of cross-continuum care often have different caseloads for case managers in different parts of the program. For example, in one organization the ratio is 45 to 1 in the ambulatory program and 25 or 30 to 1 in the program for catastrophic patients.[55]

Another way of understanding differences in case management programs is the extent of the case manager's ongoing accountability for patient management, as sum-

TABLE 6.2. COMPARISON OF INTEGRATED PRIMARY CARE CASE MANAGEMENT AND UTILIZATION MANAGEMENT.

CHARACTERISTIC	PRIMARY CARE CASE MANAGEMENT = PROACTIVE	UTILIZATION MANAGEMENT = REACTIVE
Role	Identify medically appropriate care and achieve desired patient management outcomes	Determine medical necessity by arranging prior authorization/determining medical necessity
Timing	Identify patients at risk	When patients present with illness
Focus	Continuum, including home- and community-based care	Episode of illness, typically in acute care or rehab setting
Case Load	Small number of patients (20–30)	Large numbers of patients (50–70+)
Contact with patient	Frequent (daily, weekly)	Infrequent—none

marized in Figure 6.4. Case managers are used increasingly in ambulatory care in a variety of programs sponsored by health care organizations, employers, payers, and community service agencies.[56] These models use a case manager (typically a nurse) during a particular encounter (such as an emergency room visit or ambulatory surgery or procedure) or during a specific episode (such as a workers' compensation case). Case managers in acute care and rehab settings, as well as those who manage temporary home care, typically follow patients for the duration of an episode. Primary care case management, as defined in our research, is similar to case management for patients in long-term institutional or home care in that it provides for continuity of patient management over a longer period of time—for some patients an indefinite period.

Comparison of Case Examples: Components and Degree of Integration

Care management programs for high-risk patients also span a range in terms of the components of the care process included and the extent to which components

FIGURE 6.4. SPECTRUM OF CASE MANAGEMENT MODELS IN TERMS OF EXTENT OF ONGOING ACCOUNTABILITY FOR PATIENT MANAGEMENT.

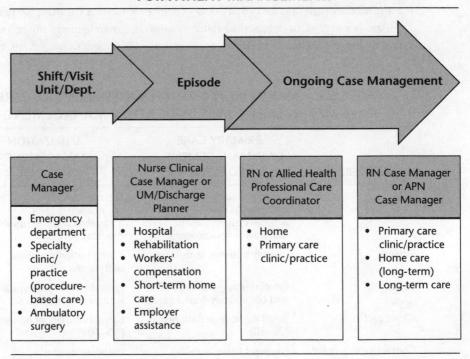

Shift/Visit Unit/Dept.	Episode	Ongoing Case Management	
Case Manager	Nurse Clinical Case Manager or UM/Discharge Planner	RN or Allied Health Professional Care Coordinator	RN Case Manager or APN Case Manager
• Emergency department • Specialty clinic/practice (procedure-based care) • Ambulatory surgery	• Hospital • Rehabilitation • Workers' compensation • Short-term home care • Employer assistance	• Home • Primary care clinic/practice	• Primary care clinic/practice • Home care (long-term) • Long-term care

are integrated into the direct care process. We identified examples that fall into the following three categories:

- Those focused on individual components of care—examples include interventions focused on patient education or compliance or provider education concerning best practices in patient management.
- Those creating a new integrated care process or model that incorporates new approaches to both care delivery and clinical management (the model that was our research focus).
- Those providing care to broad populations, extending the principles and components of all of the above models to health management (wellness, secondary prevention, and disease management, depending on the status and needs of each patient).

Figure 6.5 illustrates the spectrum of high-risk management programs. The third level—population-based management—is the future model for integrated care management. Some early case examples are beginning to emerge. We believe that this is the ultimate goal of IDNs seeking to build a system of organized care management applied to all patients.

Many programs of the first type—those that address individual components of care—can now be purchased as a service. A number are offered by the pharmaceutical industry[57, 58, 59] and include academic detailing (visits by peer physicians to individual colleagues to provide education and deliver information to change physician practice) and support services to patients provided by pharmacy benefits management companies.[60] Patient education interventions range from group

FIGURE 6.5. SPECTRUM OF HIGH-RISK MANAGEMENT PROGRAMS.

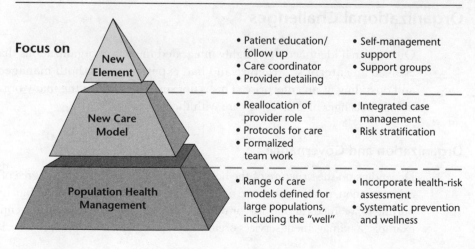

Focus on		
New Element	• Patient education/ follow up • Care coordinator • Provider detailing	• Self-management support • Support groups
New Care Model	• Reallocation of provider role • Protocols for care • Formalized team work	• Integrated case management • Risk stratification
Population Health Management	• Range of care models defined for large populations, including the "well"	• Incorporate health-risk assessment • Systematic prevention and wellness

classes to individual coaching by telephone.[7, 36, 47] These programs in some cases include specialized equipment (such as remote peak flow monitors, glucometers for assessing blood sugar levels, and home-based aerosol nebulizers) to facilitate patient personal health management and self-reporting of assessment information.[61, 62, 63] Another model of this type adds a case manager role operating outside of the practice site but leaves other elements unchanged.

Case examples that illustrate different levels of patient management are provided in Exhibits 6.3 through 6.5. Exhibit 6.3 profiles one IPA's model that provides care coordination and patient support through care coordinators who are not directly integrated into the care process.[53]

Exhibits 6.4 and 6.5 describe two different approaches to a new care model. Both include integrated primary care case management—the first employs RN case managers who partner with physicians in their assigned practice site,[20] and the second uses advanced practice nurses who assume greater responsibility for clinical management but also coordinate with PCPs and specialists for each patient.[25] These approaches use many of the same care management strategies but allocate roles and responsibilities differently among members of the care team.

Care management strategies and interventions that were initially employed in new models for high-risk patients can clearly benefit other patients. Eventually they may be applied to broad populations that are stratified according to health needs and health risk factors. Much remains to be learned about the efficacy of interventions such as primary care case management for patients with less immediate health needs, and about how to efficiently deploy proactive monitoring and follow-up for large numbers of patients; but examples are already emerging of the same approaches applied to secondary prevention in patients with identified health risk factors.[9, 10, 43]

Organizational Challenges

Our research identified only highly integrated models in organizations that had evolved an enterprise structure and had experience with both managed care and operating as an enterprise. This is not surprising, given the many organizational challenges of delivering care with the new model.

Organization and Governance

Depending on the structure of the health care organization and the degree of vertical integration, primary care case managers may be part of a corporate function (reporting to the medical director) or part of a health plan or risk-assuming entity (for example, a management services organization or independent practice association).

EXHIBIT 6.3. IPA MODEL OF HIGH-RISK PATIENT MANAGEMENT: CARE COORDINATORS NOT INTEGRATED INTO PRACTICE SITES.

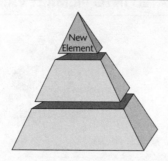

Setting/Environment
- IPA is in urban, advanced managed care market where many physicians/physician groups have separate contract affiliations with three dominant health systems.

Care Team
- Resource coordinator working out of IPA office does patient follow-up, provides connection with community services, does patient education and training, and facilitates communication between patient, physician, and community providers.
- Each managed care patient has a PCP in one of the group practice offices.
- Many physician practices have a practice nurse who performs acute episode-focused case management (for instance, patient has procedure such as hip replacement or unplanned admission).

Case Finding/Intake
- Referral comes from physicians and practice nurses or risk screening.
- Mail letter from patient's PCP and risk assessment to patients older than 65 years (includes risk of repeated hospitalization or "PRA" and adverse outcomes; also SF–36 and MHI–5).

Assess/Plan Care and Case Management
- Based on score on questionnaire, patients are triaged into three levels:
  Level 1—Provide information about activities for senior citizens, follow up every 3 months
  Level 2—Provide information about community services, future planning, and advanced directives, and follow up every month.
  Level 3—Make home visit and assess needs, provide information on community services (including personal assistance, transportation, home care, and counseling) and information and support groups; initiate and arrange referrals to community services; follow-up calls and/or visits at least monthly.

Deliver Care and Case Management
- Resource coordinator provides information on and arranges for community resources and services.
- Patients receive care from their PCPs and visiting nurses, as appropriate.

Monitor/Follow up
- Patients are instructed to call the program for assistance with the types of services covered.
- Resource coordinators make telephone calls or home visits periodically according to the level of management for each patient; they also facilitate communication between community providers and the physician practice, when the need arises.
- Resource coordinators provide regular written communications to PCPs and engage in regular telephone conversations with practice nurses and office staff.

Comments
- One challenge of this model is that only the patients covered by a particular managed care contract are eligible for the program (practices include many other patients with risk profiles that would make them eligible).

EXHIBIT 6.4. INTEGRATED MODEL OF PRIMARY CARE CASE MANAGEMENT: NURSE CASE MANAGERS INTEGRATED INTO PRIMARY CARE PRACTICE SITES.

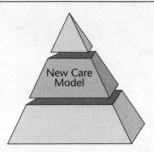

Setting/Environment
- IDN that operates a health plan in a rapidly advancing managed care market.

Care Team
- Each HMO patient has a PCP in one of the IDN practice sites.
- RN case managers work in each practice site, paired with a small number of physicians.
- Another RN assigned to each practice site is responsible for outreach to new members.
- Specialist physicians participate in patient assessments and care plan development, as appropriate to the patient's medical problems and status.

Case Finding/Intake
- Formal referrals from physicians on form that lists criteria for case management (based on levels of service and medication utilization, age, selected diagnoses for chronic or catastrophic illness, and/or status such as frail elder at risk or impaired ADL without home support); exceptions to criteria must be approved by case manager and medical director.
- New member screening performed by outreach nurse who contacts all new members to provide orientation, to assist with PCP selection, and to do risk screening.
- Population screening based on claims and clinical information to detect potential patients.
- Patients greater than 75 years of age and receiving institutionalized care (acute, rehab) are automatically reviewed for possible case management.

Assess/Plan Care and Case Management
- Primary care case managers conduct a psychosocial assessment of identified patients and perform intake as appropriate.
- PCP and primary care case manager develop care plan; primary care case manager develops case management plan.

Deliver Care and Case Management
- Primary care case managers assist with arrangements for care (both within the IDN and with community care providers).
- Patients receive most of their ambulatory care in the PCP's practice and at home (visiting nurses, as appropriate). Patients may also be referred to a specialist for consultation/assessment.
- Primary care case managers see patients in the practice site and make home visits.

Monitor/Follow up
- Primary care case managers contact patients regularly and are the first point of contact for patients. They also receive regular reports from home care providers.
- All patients are reviewed at regularly scheduled weekly clinical team meetings that include the primary care case manager, outreach nurse for the practice, PCP, clinic-based social worker, and clinical nurse reviewer.
- Primary care case managers continue to monitor patients under primary care case management when they are hospitalized. Day-to-day management, however, is handed off to an episode case manager in the hospital or to a regional case manager who follows patients in rehab and SNF sites.

EXHIBIT 6.5. INTEGRATED MODEL OF PRIMARY CARE CASE MANAGEMENT: CHRONIC DISEASE CLINIC OPERATED BY ADVANCED PRACTICE NURSES.

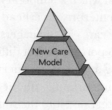

Setting/Environment
- IDN that operates its own health plan and is located in a mature managed care market.

Care Team
- Each patient has a PCP; patients enrolled in the chronic disease program still see their PCP for all but ongoing management of the chronic disease(s).
- Advanced practice nurses organized into a special clinic manage patients enrolled in the chronic disease program in conjunction with one or more specialists. They have been delegated ongoing patient management responsibility using protocols approved by a cross-specialty steering committee and the enterprise medical director. Program nurses may also consult clinical pharmacists and social workers.
- PCPs and physician specialists are notified of any changes in patient status that require reassessing care plans and receive status reports from the program nurses weekly or biweekly.
- Program nurses carry beepers and share cross-coverage so that patients and physicians can quickly reach either a patient's nurse case manager or a nurse on-call 7 days a week and 24 hours a day.

Case Finding/Intake
- Physicians refer patients using a special form. Patients admitted with designated diagnoses or picked up during new member orientation are automatically enrolled. A program nurse is available to perform in-hospital patient assessments on the same day admitted patients are referred. Other new patients receive a home or clinic visit within a few days.

Assess/Plan Care and Case Management
- Patient assessment tools and protocols guide care and case management planning including pharmacologic management and all supportive services such as home care and patient education.
- Program nurses perform patient assessments and develop patient-specific care and case management plans using standard tools and protocols. They also assist with making arrangements for IDN and community services, as necessary.

Deliver Care and Case Management
- New patients are seen weekly or biweekly in the clinic during the first six weeks. Program nurses also make home visits to see less mobile patients. In response to changes in status, they revise care and case management plans according to the protocols.
- Patients receive other routine care from their PCP and may have appointments scheduled with a specialist, as dictated by care management protocols. (The clinic performs only immunizations in the chronic disease clinic.)
- Personal health management by patients is facilitated by patient education and coaching.

Monitor/Follow up
- Program nurses assume primary responsibility for ongoing patient follow-up. They use clinic and home visits, as well as telephone conversations with patients to stay abreast of patient status and progress.
- Once patients become stabilized, program nurses can rely on telephone conversations and status reports from home care providers and require less frequent patient encounters.
- Patients and family members are encouraged to call with questions and problems at any time, are given contact information, and are instructed as to what types of situations should trigger calls. The program makes a commitment that calls will be returned within 15 minutes.
- When patients are instructed to seek care in an ED or urgent care clinic, the referring program nurse notifies staff in that location to expect the patient and collaborates with local clinicians in developing the care strategy. Program nurses also visit their patients in acute care and rehab settings when institutional care is necessary and are involved in discharge planning.

Comments
- Case managers report to the medical director of the health plan.

This makes it difficult in situations in which organizations are still in transition and the enterprise management structure is not yet fully evolved to determine the appropriate budget for absorbing the additional cost of primary care case managers. We found one example in which a temporary solution was required (the initial costs were absorbed into an enterprise overhead account) to get the program rolling.

Integrating primary care case managers to work closely with medical and administrative staff who report through a different management structure adds to the challenge of creating a working partnership. Physical location in the practice or clinic appears to be important; without proximity, it is very difficult for case managers to become integrated into the routine of the practice.[21]

In one program, case managers were originally located in a separate office building, and much of the communication between them and the practices was by telephone, fax, and occasional conferences. When office space was arranged in the practices, both physicians and case managers benefited from more informal contact and opportunities to perform "quick-response referrals" about patients who were having problems or were possible candidates for case management. In addition, monthly written reports from case managers (often unread or unfiled) could be replaced with verbal communication, resulting in short physician notes in patient charts.[22]

Clinical content (protocols for care and case management, and patient education materials) is governed by the clinical management under a medical director (typically for the enterprise or health plan). Protocol-based care is a basic tenet of every highly integrated model identified in our research; obviously, organizational process and governance to develop and deploy clinical best practices are prerequisites.

Demonstrating Value

Most organizations use pilot programs for high-risk patient management and appear to include some evaluation of outcomes (though not always formal) to prove the concept and demonstrate value. In one health care system, many physicians were initially skeptical about the value of case management and challenged the effort by referring the most difficult-to-manage patients to pilot sites. When the pilot demonstrated clearly successful outcomes for these patients, the physicians involved sold case management to their colleagues.[20]

Many of the demonstrable benefits of improved management of patients with chronic diseases are likely downstream, and trade journals still contain references to the lack of evidence of the "efficacy and cost-effectiveness" of highly integrated models for disease management.[57, 58] Organizations that have implemented these programs, however, appear to have no difficulty demonstrating sufficient value, at least to the satisfaction of the internal audience.[25, 26, 47, 64] Our research did not identify any programs that were stopped after a pilot phase. Given the growing number of these programs, formal proof of concept no longer seems as necessary (at least for high-risk patients). Despite this, pilots still make an important contribution by providing a learning laboratory on how to manage the complex new process.

The major additional direct cost of highly integrated models is the salary of primary care case managers and any other supporting staff for this new role. Despite small caseloads (depending on patient acuity, as low as 1 to 15 or 20), the payback is easily demonstrated if the annual rate of hospitalizations and other expensive care declines for even a small number of patients. The growing literature of case studies includes claims of both improved clinical management[47, 58, 61, 64, 65] and reduced costs of care.[26, 31, 47, 58, 61, 64, 65]

Engaging Physicians

The fact that highly integrated models are being implemented only in organizations with aligned enterprise and physician incentives is a large part of the answer concerning what it takes to engage physicians in new highly integrated models for care management. Even these organizations, however, work hard to achieve physician buy-in and actually roll out new models. Successful pilots with obvious value and physician "ambassadors" from pilot sites were deciding factors in several of the cases identified in our research.

Financial incentives also encourage buy-in from physicians and other key staff. For example, one health plan introduced a set of standards for extent and quality of case management and included them in the performance evaluation for the clinic administrator. One of these standards is that the clinic must have a case manager with an identified caseload of patients.[55] In another health care system, part of the physician compensation formula is now the volume of patients referred for high-risk management.[20]

Organizations identified in our research all used internal working committees of physicians and other providers in a systematic process to develop and maintain clinical protocols for their high-risk management programs.[11] The chronic conditions currently being targeted in most of these programs (that is, asthma, diabetes, and congestive heart failure) have been addressed in guidelines initiatives sponsored by the Agency for Health Care Policy and Research and medical professional societies. These provide a thorough review of evidence-based practices that serves as the starting point for developing local clinical-management strategies.

One recommended method for engaging physicians is to involve them in developing protocols to guide patient management. At one IDN, one-third of physicians have participated in a range of initiatives targeting disease management, and productivity credit is included in variable compensation. This health care system has also implemented peer-to-peer detailing and implementation councils to reinforce recommended changes in practice.[7]

Change Management

New models require substantial redesign of both practices and processes. All the organizations contacted in our research emphasized both the magnitude of the change and the resources required. Pilots perform a crucial function by road-testing the model. The most obvious and immediate changes are at care sites where new roles (such as the primary care case manager) are introduced and work tasks are reallocated. Policies and procedures covering all aspects of the new models are obviously an important first step.

Some models call for creating new practice sites or clinics oriented toward only a particular patient subgroup, such as pediatric patients with asthma or seniors enrolled in a Medicare plan. Many organizations, however, manage both regular-care patients and patients enrolled in high-risk management at the same site. With this model, front-office and clinical staff must be able to tailor the procedure to each patient, which requires first identifying patients according to their care model and then matching them with the correct procedure. (Patients were typically flagged with color labels on medical records, stickers attached to identification cards, or information included on computer registration displays.) Over time, as new care models become more differentiated, the challenge of matching patients with care model will increase.

Changes extend far beyond ambulatory care sites. As discussed in Chapter Three, one major intersection is with the access process, which functions as the front end to new models for care management. Although many high-risk patients have special telephone numbers and contact procedures, they can turn up at any telephone or care access point seeking services or information. Ideally, staff in those locations should be able to identify patients in special-care programs and notify a designated physician or case manager. In addition, triage services should be coordinated with care management models so that both clinical advice and referrals to direct care are used appropriately.[66]

The care management process intersects with other emerging enterprise processes such as managed care enrollment, capitation management, and development and deployment of best clinical practices, at a minimum. Managing enterprise processes that have so many intersections requires careful coordination with a matrix management structure to keep the pieces synchronized and processes unified in operation. (The fact that all of these are also in transition adds to the challenge.)

New models are very unfamiliar to patients and their family members; in order to participate effectively, they need to understand how their care is to be delivered, as well as learn how and where to obtain services and information.

Integrating Payer and Delivery Functions

In many health care systems, there is a trend toward merging the roles of clinical case management and utilization management. The rationale for new models of care management includes achieving cost reductions through the combination of prevention and detection, which permit resolving medical problems with less intensive interventions. Protocols aid in determining medical appropriateness for each patient, based on best practices. Thus, at some point separate processes to ensure evidence-based patient management and utilization management become redundant.

In fact, primary care case managers often receive authority to authorize and arrange services, as well as to purchase outside services (usually within some prescribed cost range). In the survey of twenty HMOs with Medicare risk contracts, 94 percent allow case managers to authorize home care, rehabilitation, and nutritional support.[38] In some models this even includes services such as skilled nursing care.[48] Health plans sometimes also authorize case managers to make exceptions to coverage rules that are in the long-term interest of managing the patient (for example, durable medical equipment or safety-related environmental changes). Rules are generally developed in advance to guide such decisions, and special procedures are developed for problematic cases ("red flags" that are clearly defined, with a protocol indicating how to proceed).

One health care system has established alternative health care, which provides services such as live-in companions, durable medical equipment, and home intravenous therapy. Case managers, with the approval of the full clinical team, can refer patients on a time-limited basis, and coverage rules are waived if the services provide "a safe and cost-effective alternative to skilled nursing facility placement or continued hospital stay."[67] Another IDN allows case managers to use alternative care benefits such as durable medical equipment and to expand use of home infusion therapy, education, and home assistance services not allowable under Medicare rules, when they permit patients to be maintained in the least restrictive, safest, and most cost-effective setting.[67]

Case managers traditionally have functioned as patient advocates, as well as coordinators for care delivery, but our research also identified a number of examples of case managers involved in some aspects of fiscal management. Policies and procedures are needed to keep these potentially conflicting roles in balance.[41, 68]

Conclusions and Predictions

Emerging models for cross-continuum care management are centered in primary care. Health care systems are first implementing new care management models for patients at high risk of decreasing functional and medical status, especially patients with one or more chronic diseases. This is the logical starting point because these patients are the least well served by the traditional, fragmented care process and because adverse outcomes for these patients place the health care system at significant financial risk when they are providing at-risk care.

New models will next be applied to secondary prevention in patients with underlying chronic illness (but at less immediate risk) and eventually more broadly in population-based management. Early adopters of integrated models for high-risk patients will probably lead the way and provide important lessons in how to apply new models efficiently, effectively, and more broadly.

Emerging process models reflect a consistent set of care management principles but span a spectrum in terms of how many interventions they include and the extent to which they are integrated into the care process. We expect process models to evolve toward increasing integration as health care systems become more integrated and gain more experience with managed care.

The role of the primary care case manager is key to new models for management of high-risk patients and to creating a coordinated and seamless process that crosses traditional boundaries of sites, settings, and disciplines. The role is universal in highly integrated models, although some organizations have carved out activities and responsibilities for subroles such as care coordinator assistant and nurse education specialist. As health care systems gain more experience, care models will be refined based on outcomes. Models for case management will be increasingly differentiated to meet the needs of broader subpopulations of patients.

Health care systems are integrating primary and specialty care in new care models for high-risk patients, but they are organizing lead and team roles for physicians differently. There is no one obviously superior approach, although fit with the enterprise's professional culture is key. Over time, the models used by particular health care systems for organizing the physician role will probably evolve differently for different patient subpopulations, based on an increasing understanding of outcomes.

The models that integrate new activities and provider roles into the care process involve substantial change. Implemented case examples today are, without exception, in organizations with highly integrated care processes and a history of governance and operation as one enterprise. Most health care systems are in earlier stages of the transition. In these systems, success will require recognizing that there are many paths, and taking bold but deliberate steps toward the vision. Keeping up with the business pressures will undoubtedly require constant pushing against organizational readiness, and accelerating change whenever possible.

Notes

1. Hoffman, C., Rice, D., and Sung, H. "Persons with Chronic Conditions: Their Prevalence and Costs." *Journal of the American Medical Association*, 1996, *276*, 1473–1479.

2. Fox, P. D., and Fama, T. "Managed Care and Chronic Illness: An Overview." In P. D. Fox and T. Fama (eds.), *Managed Care and Chronic Illness: Challenges and Opportunities*. Gaithersburg, Md.: Aspen, 1996.

3. Zitter, M. "A New Paradigm in Health Care Delivery: Disease Management." In W. E. Todd and D. Nash (eds.), *Disease Management: A Systems Approach to Improving Patient Outcomes.* Chicago: American Hospital, 1997.

4. Voelker, R. "Population-Based Medicine Merges Clinical Care, Epidemiological Techniques." *Journal of the American Medical Association,* 1994, *271,* 1301.

5. Wagner, E. H., Austin, B. T., and VonKorff, M. "Improving Outcomes in Chronic Illness." In T. Fama and P. D. Fox (eds.), *Managed Care and Chronic Illness: Challenges and Opportunities.* Gaithersburg, Md.: Aspen,1996.

6. Grower, R., Hillegass, B., and Nelson, F. "Case Management: Meeting the Needs of Chronically Ill Patients in an HMO." In P. D. Fox and T. Fama (eds.), *Managed Care and Chronic Illness: Challenges and Opportunities.* Gaithersburg, Md.: Aspen, 1996.

7. Terry, K. "Where Disease Management Is Paying Off." *Medical Economics,* 1997, *74,* 62–78.

8. Defino, T. "Keeping the Promise." *HMO Magazine,* 1995, *36,* 46–51.

9. Solberg, L. I., and others. "Using Continuous Quality Improvement to Improve Diabetes Care in Populations: The IDEAL Model." *Journal on Quality Improvement,* 1997, *23,* 581–592.

10. Christianson, J. B., and others. "Implementing Programs for Chronic Illness Management: The Case of Hypertension Services." *The Joint Commission Journal on Quality Improvement,* 1997, *23,* 593–601.

11. Kelly, J. T., and Bernard, D. B. "Clinical Practice Guidelines: Foundation for Effective Disease Management." In W. E. Todd and D. Nash (eds.), *Disease Management: A Systems Approach to Improving Patient Outcomes.* Chicago: American Hospital, 1997.

12. Sandy, L. G., and Gibson, R. "Managed Care and Chronic Care: Challenges and Opportunities." In P. D. Fox and T. Fama (eds.), *Managed Care Chronic Illness: Challenges and Opportunities.* Gaithersburg, Md.: Aspen, 1996.

13. Scott, D. E., Hu, D. J., and Hanson, I. C. "Case Management of HIV-Infected Children in Missouri." *Public Health Reports,* 1995, *110,* 355–357.

14. Graham, K., and Timney, C. B. "Continuity of Care in Addictions Treatment: The Role of Advocacy and Coordination in Case Management." *American Journal of Drug and Alcohol Abuse,* 1995, *21,* 443–462.

15. Ridgely, M. S. "Practical Issues in the Application of Case Management to Substance Abuse Treatment." *Journal of Case Management,* 1994, *3,* 132–138.

16. Erkel, E. A., Morgan, E. P., and Staples, M. A. "Case Management and Preventive Services Among Infants from Low-Income Families." *Public Health Nursing,* 1994, *11,* 352–360.

17. Piette, J., Fleishman. J. A., Mor, V., and Thompson, B. "The Structure and Process of AIDS Case Management." *Health and Social Work,* 1992, *17,* 47–56.

18. Sowell, R. L., and Grier, J. "Integrated Case Management: The Aid Atlanta Model." *Journal of Case Management,* 1995, *4,* 15–21.

19. Maddux, B. B., and Pilon, B. "Community-Based HIV+ Nurse Case Management/Primary Care Project (research report)." *AIDS Weekly,* Apr. 4, 1994, pp. 29–30.

20. Blase, N. J., and Kaufman, J. M. "Case Management in a Vertically Integrated Health Care System." *HMO Practice,* 1994, *8* (3), 110–114.

21. Anker-Unnever, L., and Netting, F. E. "Coordinated Care Partnership: Case Management with Physician Practices." *Journal of Case Management,* 1995, *4,* 3–8.

22. Netting, F. E., and Williams, F. G. "Integrating Geriatric Case Management into Primary Care Physician Practices." *Health and Social Work,* 1995, *20,* 152–155.

23. Shelton, P., Schraeder, C., Britt, T., and Kirby, R. "A Generalist Physician-Based Model for a Rural Geriatric Collaborative Practice." *Journal of Case Management,* 1994, *3,* 98–104.

24. McCulloch, D. "Learning from Diabetes: Developing Systems and Managing Care for Specific Populations." Paper presented at the National Chronic Care Consortium 1997 national conference, Transforming Care Delivery: Bridging Concepts and Practices, Minneapolis, Minnesota, Sept. 1997.

25. Brass-Mynderse, N. J. "Disease Management for Chronic Congestive Heart Failure." *Journal of Cardiovascular Nursing*, 1996, *11*, 54–62.

26. Peters, A. L., Davidson, M. B., and Ossorio, R. C. "Management of Patients with Diabetes by Nurses with Support of Subspecialists." *HMO Practice*, 1995, *9*, 8–13.

27. Lazaroff, A. "New Models for Primary Care: Geriatric Clinics and Group Clinics." Paper presented at the National Chronic Care Consortium 1997 national conference, Transforming Care Delivery: Bridging Concepts and Practices, Minneapolis, Minnesota, Sept. 1997.

28. Scott, J. C., and Robertson, B. J. "Kaiser Colorado's Cooperative Health Care Clinic: A Group Approach to Patient Care." In T. Fama and P. D. Fox (eds.), *Managed Care and Chronic Illness: Challenges and Opportunities.* Gaithersburg, Md.: Aspen, 1996.

29. Wagner, E., Austin, B., and Galvin, M. S. "Chronic Care Clinics." Paper presented at the second annual invitational conference of the American Association of Health Plans Foundation, Chronic Care Initiatives in HMOs, Washington, D.C., Nov. 1996.

30. Simmons, J. "Patients Taking Control of Diabetes." *Healthplan*, 1997, *38*, 56–63.

31. Lumsdon, K. "Working Smarter, Not Harder." *Hospitals & Health Networks*, 1995, *69*, 27–31.

32. Scott, J., Beck, A., and Venohr, I. "Cooperative Health Care Clinic." Paper presented at the second annual invitational conference of the American Association of Health Plans Foundation, Chronic Care Initiatives in HMOs, Washington, D.C., Nov. 1996.

33. Michaels, C., and others. *Risk Identification: Exploring a Conceptual Framework and Identifying Implementation Issues.* Bloomington, Minn.: National Chronic Care Consortium, 1995.

34. Aliberti, E., and others. *Identifying High-Risk Medicare HMO Members: A Report from the HMO Workgroup on Care Management.* Washington, D.C.: Group Health Foundation, 1996.

35. Lopez, L. "Improving Care for the Frail Elderly." *Healthplan*, 1996, *37*, 39–46.

36. Matheson, P. A., and Fallon, L. F. "Nurse Telephone Screening of New Medicare HMO Members: A Pilot Program." *HMO Practice*, 1996, *9*, 14–18.

37. Major, M. J. "Managed Care and Case Management: The Dynamic Duo of the Future." *Managed Healthcare*, Aug. 1996, pp. 28–32.

38. Pacala, J. F., and others. "Case Management of Older Adults in Health Maintenance Organizations." *Journal of the American Geriatrics Society*, 1995, *43*, 538–542.

39. Kane, R. L., Illston, L. H., and Miller, N. A. "Qualitative Analysis of the Program of All-Inclusive Care of the Elderly (PACE)." *The Gerontologist*, 1992, *32*, 771–780.

40. Wolfe, G. S., and Smith, D. S. *Standards of Practice for Case Management.* Little Rock, Ark.: Case Management Society of America, 1995, p. 12.

41. Murer, C., and Brick, L. *The Case Management Sourcebook: A Guide to Designing and Implementing a Centralized Case Management System.* New York: McGraw-Hill, 1997.

42. Nelson, S. Z., Mensing, C., Baines, B., and Smith, J. "An Integrated Continuum of Care." *HMO Practice*, 1995, *9*, 40–43.

43. Levknecht, L., Schriefer, J., Schriefer, J., and Maconis, B. "Combining Case Management, Pathways, and Report Cards for Secondary Cardiac Prevention." *Joint Commission Journal on Quality Improvement*, 1997, *23*, 162–174.

44. Schneider, B., and others. *Conceptualizing, Implementing, and Evaluating Extended Care Pathways.* Bloomington, Minn.: National Chronic Care Consortium, 1995.

45. Pacala, J. F., and others. *Case Management in Health Maintenance Organizations: Final Report.* Washington, D.C.: Group Health Foundation, 1996.

46. Roussel, H. M. "Drug Firm Helps Pharmacists Help Patients." *On Managed Care,* 1997, *2,* 6.

47. Grahl, C. "Implementing the New Asthma Guidelines." *Managed Healthcare,* 1997, *7,* 56–61.

48. Gerson, V. "The Changing Face of Case Management." *Healthplan,* 1997, *38,* 77–80.

49. Collier, P., and Early, A. "A Team Approach to Geriatric Case Management." *Journal of Case Management,* 1995, *4,* 66–70.

50. Bilodeau, A. "The Heart of the Matter." *Healthplan,* 1996, *37,* 57–61.

51. Balas, E. A., and others. "Electronic Communication with Patients: Evaluation of Distance Medicine Technology." *Journal of the American Medical Association,* 1997, *278,* 152–159.

52. Macko, P., and others. "The Social HMOs Meeting the Challenge of Integrated Team Care Coordination." *Journal of Case Management,* 1995, *4,* 102–106.

53. Levinson, W., and Moore, R. "Integrating Case Management into an IPA." Paper presented at the second annual invitational conference of the American Association of Health Plans Foundation, Chronic Care Initiatives in HMOs, Washington, D.C., Nov. 1996.

54. Grower, R. "Care Coordination in the Primary Care Clinic Setting." Paper presented at the second annual invitational conference of the American Association of Health Plans Foundation, Chronic Care Initiatives in HMOs, Washington, D.C., Nov. 1996.

55. Aliotta, S. L. "Components of a Successful Case Management Program." In P. D. Fox and T. Fama (eds.), *Managed Care and Chronic Illness: Challenges and Opportunities.* Gaithersburg, Md.: Aspen, 1996.

56. Donovan, M. R. "Introduction to Outpatient Case Management." In American Hospital Association (ed.), *Outpatient Case Management: Strategies for a New Reality.* Chicago: American Hospital,1997.

57. Hensley, S. "A Difficult Pill to Swallow: Hard Sell on Disease Management Raises Eyebrows." *Modern Healthcare,* 1997, *27,* 34–35.

58. Peterson, C. "Disease Management: A Team Approach to Chronic Care." *HMO Practice,* 1995, *36,* 38–47.

59. Bernard, S. "The Roles of Pharmaceutical Companies in Disease Management." In W. E. Todd and D. Nash (eds.), *Disease Management: A Systems Approach to Improving Patient Outcomes.* Chicago: American Hospital, 1996.

60. Muir, L. "Disease Management." *Hospitals & Health Networks,* 1997, *71,* 24–30.

61. Stevens, M. A., and Weiss-Harrison, A. "A Program for Children with Asthma." *HMO Practice,* 1993, *7,* 91–93.

62. Ahring, K. K., Ahring, B. P., Joyce, C., and Farid, N. R. "Telephone Modem Access Improves Diabetes Control in Those with Insulin-Requiring Diabetes." *Diabetes Care,* 1992, *15,* 971–975.

63. Lester, J. A., and Breudigam, M. "Nurse Triage Telephone Centers: Key to Demand Management Strategy." *NAHAM Management Journal,* Spring 1996, pp. 13–34.

64. Terry, K. "Where Disease Management Is Paying Off." *Medical Economics,* 1997, *74,* 62–78.

65. Beck, A., and others. "A Randomized Trial of Group Outpatient Visits for Chronically Ill Older HMO Members: Cooperative Health Care Clinic." *Journal of the American Gerontological Society,* 1997, *45,* 543–549.

66. Kinney, N. "If You Treat It, the Savings Will Come." *Managed Healthcare,* 1997, *7,* 37–40.

67. Fama, T., and Fox, P. D. "Beyond the Benefit Package." *HMO Practice,* 1996, *9,* 179–181.

68. Banja, J., and others. "The Ethics Summit: Ethical Accountabilities for Case Management." In *Upward Bound: Case Management Society's Seventh Annual Conference.* Little Rock, Ark.: Case Management Society of America, 1997.

CHAPTER SEVEN

CROSS-CONTINUUM CARE MANAGEMENT: INFORMATION MANAGEMENT CHALLENGES

Jane Metzger

The information challenges of the new cross-continuum care models described in Chapter Six are daunting at any level but especially for integrated systems that provide cross-continuum care. We have yet to find a single organization that is very far down the road toward meeting the challenges with information technology. In fact in many cases, the telephone is still the major communication mode for cross-site and interdisciplinary coordination, and primary care case managers organize their work using a personal calendar book and a three-ring, loose-leaf binder with separate tabs for each patient.

Improving information management is critical to accomplishing many of the business objectives for the new process. It will also be a prerequisite to extending the care management principles and process to large numbers of patients and to patient subpopulations beyond those with severe chronic disease. This chapter reviews the information management challenges and profiles the characteristics of solutions.

A Layered Look at the Challenges

Opportunities for improving information management in support of cross-continuum care management can be described at three levels:

- *Support to the role of the primary care case manager.* This role is totally new in the primary care setting, and it is key to both continuity of care and teamwork. As an initial step, the case manager's job can be made more efficient and effective by providing fairly basic assistance with information management.
- *Support to primary care practices and clinics that are involved with high-risk patient management programs.* Eventually most health care systems will widely implement patient care computer systems in ambulatory care sites. Targeting initial assistance to sites that are involved with the new care management model for high-risk patients is an appealing strategy.
- *Enterprisewide support in health care systems that include high-risk patient management programs.* Many information linkages will be required across the enterprise to support continuity of care and the desired close coordination. There are opportunities, however, for stepwise progress with incremental improvements.

Looking at information challenges in these levels provides a useful framework for devising incremental solutions that first meet basic system requirements and then introduce more advanced support. It also helps in constructing a migration strategy.

Primary Care Case Manager

Basic Workflow Management. Primary care case managers are quite mobile, and their workday consists of a series of communications, coordination tasks, and patient interactions. Workflow management tools can replace the personal calendar book and three-ring notebook with a more effective means for keeping track of and accomplishing these many discrete tasks.

Case managers need to track their own schedules for team meetings and patient visits, as well as the schedules of their patients. Tools for recording schedules and frequent updates to them and the ability to access a consolidated view for any given day can save considerable time and improve time management. (Eventually, direct access to enterprise scheduling applications will simplify some coordination tasks for the case manager and eliminate the need for redundant recording of some appointments.)

In addition to attending scheduled meetings and encounters with patients, case managers make frequent follow-up telephone calls to patients, family members, and extended-care team members. Tracking and ensuring that they all attend to every follow-up task is extremely difficult. Workflow management and computer applications can provide increasing levels of support to this part of the role in the following ways:

- Self-prompting reminders can be set by the case manager for predetermined times and displayed and tracked on task lists until completion.

- Tasks can be automatically generated from case management plans (typically including many coordination tasks to be completed, as well as a plan for timed patient follow-up).

- Requests from other members of the care team (such as the primary physician) can be integrated into task lists.

- Protocol-based prompts can be used (see the upcoming section "Opportunities for Decision Support").

Even the basic level of self-prompting makes a big difference, because case managers spend so much of their time on these tasks.

Documentation. Documentation tasks for primary care case managers include both case management records for their assigned patients and notes concerning all interactions with patients, family members, and the care team.

For case management records, standard forms are typically used for record keeping on paper, and templates are important to guide electronic information capture. At a minimum, these forms and templates include risk-screening instruments (if performed by the case manager), intake forms, assessments, and case management plans. Forms and templates are tailored to diagnosis or condition, patient stratification, and other characteristics, such as age group. For complex patients, both paper forms and electronic templates are unwieldy and must be combined and substantially customized. (See the upcoming section "Opportunities for Decision Support.")

Often the same information ends up being recorded over and over again. Case managers must copy information about the care plan from the patient's medical record to guide coordination and follow-up portions of the case management plan. As more key patient information is captured electronically and can be integrated into case manager support, redundant documentation should be reduced.

Depending on the organization's medical record practices, some case management documentation may also be filed in a patient's medical record. At a minimum this usually includes the intake assessment (or a summary thereof) and periodic patient status assessments. This requirement is met in paper records by filing duplicate copies or preparing status summaries for physicians that are subsequently filed in medical records. Integrated electronic health records that contain comprehensive documentation of care and case management will meet these needs for broader access to information for all members of the care team. As an interim solution, access to common electronic case management records among the case management staff can facilitate cross-coverage among case managers and program supervision.

Case managers also document their many telephone consultations with patients and others. Some of these can be guided by templates (examples are provided in the scenarios in Chapter Eight). Keeping a record of all interactions is important. An electronic history of patient interactions that integrates both structured documentation and telephone notes is extremely useful in ongoing patient management, especially if it can be viewed in different ways (time view, type of interaction, or patient interactions only).

Communication. A major role of the primary care case manager is to facilitate communication within the care team and ensure that various members have timely status updates appropriate to their roles. This function is time-consuming and can be improved in several ways.

Much communication occurs by telephone. When the task at hand is to transfer information or ask a fairly straightforward question, electronic mail is quicker and much more effective than playing "phone tag." In some of the programs identified in our research, case managers who currently rely on the telephone viewed the possibility of electronic mail as something approaching Nirvana. Electronic mail connections with the primary physicians with whom they work were at the top of the wish list, followed by links to other care team members, such as specialist physicians. Similar connections with the extended care team, including visiting nurses and episode case managers in hospitals and other institutional settings, would make routine communication with them easier and more efficient. (Medical directors and case manager supervisors with whom we spoke, however, cautioned against viewing electronic mail as a total solution, because many care management situations require more than a "virtual dialogue.")

Case managers usually maintain paper records of contact information, such as telephone numbers and listings for patients, internal service sites and providers, and community providers. Basic tools for organizing and accessing this information would be a boon. Shared records within a case or patient management program or even within the enterprise are better still, because much of the information has broader applicability.

Correspondence is another opportunity for improvement. Case managers correspond frequently with community providers and payers. Word processing with letter templates, which include automatic incorporation of contact and patient-specific information, offers the combined advantages of efficient document preparation for the case manager and an electronic record for subsequent retrieval. (Ideally, correspondence is integrated with the electronic history of other types of patient-related communications and interactions.)

As discussed in Chapter Six, regularly scheduled team meetings are a common feature of highly integrated models for high-risk patients. Case managers have the most frequent contact with patients and thus are the logical team member to organize status information and other notes for discussion. This function is quite similar to assembling information for nursing end-of-shift reporting in hospitals—the ideal is an electronic summary listing of patients that includes appropriate information about recent interactions and status, and this is a good long-term goal for computer support. Probably more feasible in the short term, however, is an increasing ability to assemble relevant notes and communications as more information is captured electronically and becomes accessible for this purpose. (An example of how this might work is provided in Chapter Eight.)

Ambulatory Care Site

Patient Intake and Orientation. Responsibility for new-member orientation often lies with primary care case managers in ambulatory practices or clinics. As discussed in Chapter Three, orientation is sometimes delegated to triage nurses in access centers; in some organizations this is an enterprise-level function. The information challenges are the same, although the users and access locations differ depending on how this function is organized.

To perform risk screening and other orientation, providers should identify new members as soon as possible. Some organizations target patient subpopulations defined by age (for example, over sixty-five years of age) or health plan (for example, all enrolled members of a Medicare plan). The process can be further assisted by the following:

- Automatic mailing of orientation materials to identified new members, including risk screening instruments, as appropriate.

- Workflow management to support response tracking and telephone outreach to administer a risk-screening instrument and to follow up with nonrespondents to mail surveys

- Automated identification of patients with incomplete orientation status (for example, listings of patients with no PCP selection recorded)

- Recording of patient responses to telephone-administered surveys, and tools for translating patient-reported information into electronic form

- Automated analysis of risk-screening information and stratification of patients according to scores

A goal of many programs that utilize telephone-based outreach is to perform all orientation activities during one patient contact. Accomplishing this efficiently for large numbers of patients will require most of the capabilities just listed. In addition, staff need the capability to assist with PCP selection and, when risk screening is involved, to triage and schedule patients for immediate services, as warranted.

Despite considerable efforts to orient new members on enrollment, it is inevitable that some will call or arrive for services before orientation can be completed. An ideal for the future is for staff at telephone and service access locations to be able to identify patient orientation status and accomplish requisite orientation activities.

Care Planning. The most basic information challenge in care planning is to assemble the available information for each patient and organize it to facilitate review by the care team. For patients with chronic disease, the ability to examine trends in pertinent status information (such as measurements and diagnostic results), singly and in combination with information on medications and other interventions, is the highest priority. Also important are risk-screening results (for new patients) and the ability to review and integrate functional status information and patient self-monitoring.

Care and case management planning are interrelated. A goal in many programs is a structured, comprehensive assessment encompassing both health and psychosocial status rather than separate, and in some cases redundant, patient assessments and care and case management planning. A more coordinated approach is achieved by scheduling some or all patient encounters with the care team as a group, and by holding regularly scheduled team meetings. Achieving similar coordination of the information tasks requires integrated templates incorporating all available information.

Implementing protocols for care and case management is complicated by the fact that complex patients have multiple chronic problems and other unique factors to address. Combining and customizing care protocols is unwieldy either on paper or in system templates that are not designed to be combined and customized based on patient-specific information. Ultimate solutions that facilitate both care planning and documentation will rely on clinical decision support to manage this complexity. (Opportunities for decision support are discussed later in this chapter.)

Both care and case management plans are structured as time-based plans (as opposed to reflecting only current interventions). They are similar to the pathways format that is being implemented for some hospital inpatients in that they incorporate explicit goals with respect to objective assessments and function. Even in the absence of tools to facilitate developing care plans from model plans or protocols, recording medical management goals and interventions electronically is a high priority both to support continuity of care and to build databases for practice analysis. Recording the case management plan is also important for continuity of care among case managers but a lower priority for enterprisewide access.

Another important reason for electronic capture of both care and case management plans is the relative ease of tracking and documenting progress toward goals and compliance with interventions. This is also the only realistic way to capture structured information on variances to be incorporated in practice analysis.

Enterprise Scheduling/Access to Care. In the highly integrated models identified in our research, care and case management are performed from the practice site. Service coordination and patient compliance monitoring are greatly facilitated if case managers and other staff can obtain a consolidated view of appointments for their patients, book new appointments for enterprise services at the practice site and other locations, and review encounter histories to verify service completion.

Enterprise

Patient Registry. Traditional registration systems usually maintained information on a patient's PCP and possibly also on the primary location of the patient's medical record. Initial experience with new care models for high-risk patients clearly shows a need for maintaining additional information in a patient registry.

For immediate patient management purposes, the following information should be maintained and accessible:

- Patient care model (likely to include a diagnosis or diagnostic grouping and level of care and case management such as "CHF-Level 4"; for some patients the care model of "routine care" or employer-based program will be appropriate)
- Date of enrollment in current care model
- Primary care team: primary physician and case manager (as applicable)
- Primary extended care team: specialist physicians, dietitians, social workers, and so on
- Primary family contact person
- Patient current location—home, rehabilitation site, hospital, or other facility—and status
- Current responsible care team (if different from primary team)

As patients are followed for longer periods, changes will occur in all of this information, and it will be important to retain patient histories as well as information on their current status.

A patient registry will become increasingly important as new care management principles are applied more broadly. Ideally, at least basic information on care model and responsible case manager and primary physician is available at any telephone or physical access point in the care system. The next logical extension is to provide information on immediate contact (or notification) procedures and contact information, including cross-coverage for case managers and primary physicians during off hours. Enterprise staff will need this information to respond appropriately when patients call or come in for services.

Many of the examples identified in our research integrate management of high-risk patients with that of other patients in ambulatory practice sites. A patient registry will help providers and front-office staff identify patients assigned to different care models and follow appropriate procedures when patients call or arrive for services. The need for this capability will grow as the number of care models increases.

Population Screening. Scanning available databases of electronic patient information to identify patients who could benefit from more intensive care management is practiced or planned in all the sites with new care models identified in our research. Population screening turns out to be an important adjunct to new-member screening and professional referrals, and it offers the possibility of identifying candidates for intensive care management early in the process. The ability to screen the population is a function of the extent of common databases and the ability to link services for a patient across sites and settings of care.

Typically, decision rules are used to screen patient data. Because claims are often the best source available, decision rules focus on utilization patterns, accrued service costs, and to some degree, the diagnostic coding incorporated in claims. Laboratory results and pharmacy databases are sometimes used but are obviously more limited in the scope of patient services that can be reviewed. As more clinical information becomes available in enterprise databases, it should be possible to use clinically based decision rules for earlier detection of patients with changes in health status.

Patients identified through population screening are potential candidates for high-risk management programs. To assist case managers and others in further evaluating individual patients, listings of referrals and other services for the time period scanned are desirable.

Continuity of Care. Information access is critical to achieving continuity of care between individual care providers and across the sites and settings of care. When patient care computer systems have advanced to the point described in a study on computer-based patient records by the Institute of Medicine,[1] health care systems will be approaching the ideal. In the meantime, however, progress on this front will be incremental.

The program managers interviewed during our research stressed two types of information as being most critical to continuity of care: the ability to recognize patients in a special care model and obtain contact information for their case manager and primary physician, and access to the current care plan for the patient. The need for this information suggests areas for early focus in improving information access. The first is considerably easier to accomplish than the second, however.

Planned transitions between care settings, such as a patient hospital discharge to home, provide opportunities for deliberate transfers of information to accompany (or even precede) the transfer of care responsibility. Predetermining what information should be transferred is one of the principles underlying the Extended Care Pathway that is being implemented by members of the National Chronic Care Consortium.[2] This strategy is another way to ensure that even paper-based information supports continuity of care and will also identify critical information needs for system migration planning.

In IDNs with emerging enterprise processes for access to care, some of the care management functions, such as telephone follow-up of high-risk patients, are being delegated to triage nurses in access centers. The information requirements of this process are reviewed in Chapter Four and are not repeated here, except the point that continuity of care requires a two-way exchange of triage notes, other telephone notes, and messages with physicians and primary care case managers throughout the enterprise.

Opportunities for Decision Support

Once sufficient electronic data become available and providers routinely access computer systems as they perform patient management tasks, there are many opportunities for clinical decision support to improve efficiency and effectiveness.

Case Finding and Intake. Decision support can assist staff in accomplishing tasks relating to new-member orientation and intake in a number of ways:

- Automated identification of new members, and preparation and mail-out of requisite orientation materials (deficiencies in the capture of enrollment information will be a gating factor in success)

- Automated identification of potential patients for intensive care models by real-time or frequent scanning of claims and patient clinical information

- Protocol-based prompting of case managers and other providers who administer risk-screening instruments, combined with real-time scoring and patient risk stratification, to identify the appropriate response to the information obtained

Each of these methods promises to increase the timeliness, efficiency, and consistency of task completion, and they will likely evolve in the order shown.

Assess Health and Plan Care. Decision support is urgently needed to accomplish business objectives such as providing appropriate care management to each patient and a single standard of care in the enterprise. Realistically, some decision support will be a prerequisite for consistent application of care and case management protocols.

The ideal data flow and contributions of decision support are pictured in Figure 7.1 and include the following components:

- Contributions of patient assessment information from various sources

- Incorporation of information on current patient status and stratification (care model)

- Algorithm-based tools for conducting current assessments and developing customized patient management strategies

- Prompts to responsible care givers to follow up with patients or reevaluate care management strategies based on rules-based review of new assessment information

Simple protocols in a pathway format will suffice in some care situations. Algorithm-based tools that incorporate decision trees and branching based on accumulated information are required for complex patients, however. Ideally, both medical care and case management planning are supported by rules-based decision support that triggers a prompt or message when significant changes are detected in new patient assessment information.

High-risk patients are assessed frequently, and the process depicted in Figure 7.1 is dynamic. Alerting physicians and primary care case managers when new assessment information becomes available can greatly facilitate timely responses to updates. The scenarios in Chapter Eight provide several examples of how this type of decision support could assist the care team, as well as an example of algorithm-based tools for case management planning.

Our research identified one organization, ScrippsHealth, that is implementing computer-based decision support to care and case management planning. At ScrippsHealth, nurse case managers are also advanced practice nurses. They utilize complex algorithms for pharmacologic management of chronic congestive heart

FIGURE 7.1. SCHEMATIC DIAGRAM OF DECISION SUPPORT APPLIED TO ASSESSMENT AND CARE MANAGEMENT PLANNING.

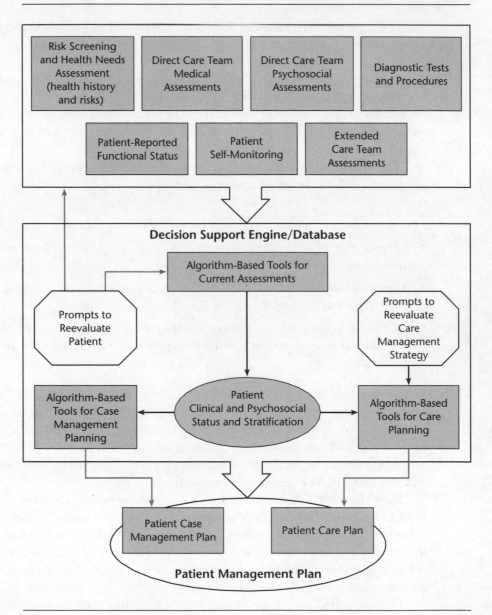

failure and other problems to construct care plans for each patient, using a decision database program developed jointly with a vendor.[3] Patient assessment data are entered into the computer program. For dietary and lipid management, the nurse case managers utilize guidelines with a decision tree and branching to prescribe type of diet, applicability and dosage for cholesterol-lowering agents, and follow-up care. Whenever new assessment information is entered, the decision support rules suggest changes in therapy based on functional status, blood pressure, laboratory results, report of symptoms, exercise testing, and response to medications.

Health plan coverages differ in several significant ways that affect care management. When up-to-date information on patient eligibility and coverage is available, decision support can make further contributions in assisting the care team to work within a plan's established rules and boundaries:

- Prompts to notify responsible care sites and care managers when patient enrollment status changes

- Prompts to notify care managers when patient eligibility and coverage changes in a way that affects the current care management strategy and scheduled services

- Support for closed formularies and rules concerning covered services and providers through the display of choices based on covered options

- Prompts when planned interventions are not covered or have financial implications for the patient

Patient enrollment is always subject to change (until recently as frequently as every thirty days for Medicare enrollees), and health plan coverage rules are a moving target. Decision support offers a coordinated way to assist providers in doing the right things in the right way for their patients. (Realistically, progress in applying computer decision support to this problem will be slow and incremental.)

Monitor and Follow-Up. One major challenge of patient follow-up is tracking to ensure that planned interventions occur and to keep informed of unplanned interventions. Depending on the extent of enterprise applications and databases, there are several types of opportunities to assist the care team by flagging occurrences that warrant follow-up:

- For scheduled interventions that involve enterprise providers and care locations, notifying designated care managers when services are delayed or canceled and when patients fail to show up for care

- Notifying care managers when patients request or arrive for emergency or urgent services at any location in the enterprise
- For medications, notifying care managers when patients fail to pick up prescribed medications and refills (likely to require electronic linkages with community pharmacies)

Some organizations attempt these types of procedures without much automation; it is difficult and labor-intensive but not impossible. The most common example identified in our research is real-time notification of patient arrival in an emergency room or subsequent forwarding of a copy of the ED report, with urgent notification when a patient is admitted from the emergency room. (This requires a patient registry or other mechanism for flagging patients under care management and identifying responsible care providers.) Decision support can make these types of procedures feasible for a broad range of services and for large numbers of patients, including those assigned to a routine care model.

New Types of Information

Emerging models require the capture and use of new types of information. Much of this information is important for both individual patient management and outcomes analysis.

Patient-Provided Information. Patients are being asked to report certain types of information used at various stages of care management:

- Information used to screen for participation in high-risk management programs. This can be obtained by patient self-reporting on survey instruments or recorded by staff who interview patients by telephone or in person.
- Periodically reported information on patient functional status.[4, 5] This is used both for assessing individual patient progress and in outcomes analysis.[6]
- Patient personal health management contracts. Patients collaborate with their care teams to develop an agreement about goals and self-management activities.
- Patient assessment information (such as peak flow values and blood sugars) obtained in self-monitoring. Care providers use this information to provide a more complete record of trends in patient status.

All of this information must be retained for subsequent reference. Most of it is managed on paper today, although many health care systems hope to migrate to electronic capture and eventual integration into the patient electronic health record. When this is possible, patient-reported information will have to be identified to differentiate it from observations and assessments by clinicians.

Case Management Acuity. Managing caseloads of primary care case managers will require an acuity-based system for rating the relative intensity of case management, very similar to acuity weightings used for nursing staffing in the acute care environment. Support to caseload management may be possible in increments based on the increasing availability of electronic information and automated analysis, including basic tools for using patient risk stratification, diagnosis, and interventions in the case management plan to calculate acuity for individual patients; automated calculation of acuity based on assessment information and the case management plan; and acuity-based caseload analysis and reporting. Tools of this sort will become increasingly important as new care models employing primary care case managers are extended to broader patient populations. Patient case management acuity will also be useful as one measure of severity in outcomes analysis.

Patient Education. Empowering patients in self-management is a core principle of new models. Performing and tracking patient education in a coordinated way involves new information management challenges of several different kinds.

For individual patient education, case managers, physicians, and nurse education specialists all need access to materials in each setting where they perform education and coaching. Typically, education is customized to each patient according to the chronic condition targeted, specific care management strategy (especially medications and self-management), capacity for self-management, and (if necessary) reading level. The ability to customize materials and handouts is key.

Education is an intervention included in most case management plans. Because it must often be repeated or reinforced through coaching, additional case management interventions are often included in the plan to allow time for this activity. Both completion and patient comprehension need to be documented each time a case manager or education specialist delivers education or coaching. Ideally documentation includes a copy of the actual materials and handouts so that case managers and other care team members can answer subsequent patient questions and review specific portions with the patient.

Group sessions for support and education are also part of a number of identified models. Case managers and other responsible providers must be able to identify participating patients and track their participation in patient encounter histories. Recording appointments for future group sessions allows a case manager to coordinate other appointments and reinforce patient compliance during follow-up. For staff responsible for running group encounters, ease of scheduling and recording attendance for group sessions is important (ideally linked to documentation of patient interactions).

External Care Team. Case managers often interact with home- and community-based care providers who are not employees of the health care system. To schedule and coordinate services with these external providers, case managers need access to information on community resources. In addition, records of service appointments with external providers ideally should be integrated with other scheduled services for patients so that case managers can obtain a composite view of scheduled interventions and monitor and document completion.

Periodically, case managers also interact with visiting nurses and other external providers to follow up on patient progress. Either electronic messaging or direct access to status reports and assessments would facilitate this communication and permit assessment information from the home and community care sites to be incorporated into outcomes analysis.

Enhancing Patient Communications

Telephone and the Internet are providing new ways for patients to obtain information and make connections with their care team that may substitute for in-person care encounters and empower patients in self-management.

Telephone Care. The telephone is being used in many innovative ways in the management of high-risk patients:

- Modem connections are being used to transmit assessment information such as blood pressure, blood sugar, and peak flow readings from home monitors.[7,8]
- Interactive voice response is being used to obtain patient-reported assessment measurements and functional status self-reporting.[9,10]
- Computer-controlled digitized speech is being used to conduct virtual dialogues with patients in which they provide information to their care team or obtain remote counseling on topics such as medication compliance and self-management behavior.[9]

Patient acceptance and emerging evidence concerning the effectiveness of these uses will lead to their wider application.[7,9]

The Internet. The Internet revolution is also affecting care and self-management of high-risk patients. Both use rates and research with patient focus groups indicate that patients are positively disposed to on-line access and that it can meet information and support the needs of the chronically ill.[7,11–14]

Health care systems are either sponsoring or facilitating patient access to on-line information and support groups.[15–20] Emerging applications include on-line submission of assessment information and functional status assessments.[21,22] (The scenarios in Chapter Eight include some examples of how the Internet can facilitate patient connections with the health care system and with Web-based information resources.)

Equipping Patients. Not all patients are equipped with the necessary technology to take advantage of emerging opportunities for distance connections. Although the telephone is available nationally in more than 90 percent of households, access in some communities is as low as 60 percent. Internet access is far less universal: as few as 14 percent of the population are estimated to have access.[23]

Some health care systems have experimented with equipping particularly at-risk patients with distance technology. For example, as part of one program for disadvantaged patients, a health care system provided cellular telephones to patients requiring frequent follow-up.[24] In another experimental program, patients with chronic diseases have been given personal computers for use at home to access information on self-management and community resources, participate in support groups, and communicate easily with their care team.[12, 25]

Distance technology is likely to become much more universal in the future through cable networks and public service networks with two-way, high-speed capacities and in-home devices such as "smart televisions."[22, 23]

Outcomes

Evidence-based care management is a core principle of new models for patient management, and experience-based care management a long-term goal. Most organizations, however, face an enormous gap in their ability to analyze practice information in the way they would like, and a significant time lag before they will be in a position to do so.

Scope of Analysis. Although there is general agreement about the importance of outcomes measurement and management, this aspect of new programs is still in its infancy because of difficulties in defining useful measures of value and obtaining the necessary information.

An important first step is defining the outcomes of interest. Outcomes are defined differently depending on their impetus and use. One taxonomy for organizing the many possible measures for new care management models includes clinical, economic, organizational, behavioral, and quality outcomes.[5] Exhibit 7.1 provides examples of measures for each type of outcome.

In many organizations, claims data are still the best (and sometimes only) source of information for tracking care management activities. For this reason, the most

EXHIBIT 7.1. EXAMPLES OF OUTCOME MEASURES
FOR NEW CARE MANAGEMENT MODELS.

Clinical*	• Patients with (specified) complication or (specified) acute episode per (specified) time period • Average number of (specified) complications per patient per time period • Patients attaining (specified) functional status within (specified) time period following (specified) intervention or (specified) acute episode • Patients at (specified) physiologic status standard • Patients receiving recommended preventive interventions within (specified) time standard • Patients receiving recommended follow-up interventions within (specified) time standard • Patients receiving recommended follow-up interventions within (specified) time standard • Patients receiving treatment within (specified) time standard after diagnosis
Economic*	• Costs of hospitalization per patient per year • Costs of urgent or emergency care per patient per year • Utilization of emergency care per patient per year • Referrals to specialist per patient per year
Organizational*	• Members receiving risk screening within (specified) time standard following enrollment • Members receiving risk screening before first health encounter • New member orientation to care model within (specified) time standard following enrollment in care model • Response time for patient telephone calls to care management team • Physician referrals to high-risk management program • High-risk patients with intake assessment within (specified) time standard following enrollment in care model • Disease stage at enrollment in care model
Behavioral*	• Patients achieving self-management goals • Patient compliance with (specified) care and treatment • Patient compliance with medications prescribed • Patients achieving recommended lifestyle modification • Provider compliance with (specified) recommended care management interventions • Patients receiving recommended (specified) education or coaching
Quality*	• Population achievement of (specified) level of functional status • Patient-reported quality of life • Patient satisfaction with quality of care • Provider satisfaction with quality of care delivered • Patients receiving (specified) standard of care

* Note: All for severity-adjusted specified patient subpopulations

commonly employed outcomes encountered in our research were economic ones, such as avoided hospitalizations and costs of care. These measures have proven useful in demonstrating the ability to offset increased costs of case management and other interventions, but they do little to address the longer-term goal of continuous practice improvement.

The report card movement is providing external stimulus to examining defined outcomes of new care management models for purchasers and consumers. Because health care systems have so much progress to make in electronic information capture, industry report cards may provide some of the impetus for early focus on some types of information. Initial measures for a few chronic diseases focused on secondary prevention (for example, foot examinations in patients with diabetes). More recently, organizations such as the National Committee for Quality Assurance, the Foundation for Accountability, and Health Care Financing Administration have been adding measures focusing on population management, including populations defined by disease burden and by age.[5, 26-28] A new element in many measures is patient-reported functional status. Many health care systems are already collecting this information for patient management; inclusion in mandated reporting measures underlines the importance of capturing the information electronically and providing access to functional status in conjunction with other patient-specific information.

Special Challenges. As mentioned earlier, definitions are still evolving as health care systems attempt to put in place systems and processes for meeting the information needs of outcomes analysis. Two challenges deserve special mention, because substantial progress will be required before outcomes information can be put to use in evidence-based care.

For many outcomes relating to chronic disease and wellness, the useful period of analysis will be the year. This is especially true for economic outcomes relating to service utilization and cost. Additional constructs will be required, however, for examining processes and clinical outcomes within stages of care management, such as an episode of illness, care, or disease.[29, 30] When defined in the context of cross-continuum care management, the episode is usually more than an individual encounter, but it is not necessarily indefinite. Unfortunately, definition requires grappling with how to define nonoverlapping periods of care, beginning with problem identification or initiation of care management responsibility and ending with problem resolution or transfer of care management. Different definitions of episodes may in fact be required for examining different types of outcomes. Once episodes have been defined, a further challenge is how to align information management to provide a clear tracking of documentation of services and episodes.

Another critical challenge lies in defining meaningful subpopulations of patients for analysis. At a minimum this requires information on diagnosis, stage or severity of disease, and complicating factors. For certain types of outcomes, further distinctions will be required. For example, case management acuity may be needed to examine effectiveness of different case management models, or a rating of patient self-management capability to compare effectiveness of different approaches to patient education and coaching.

The increasing interest of government, business, and consumer groups in health outcomes information is focusing a great deal of attention on obtaining reliable and meaningful information. This movement will push the whole industry to develop and implement new definitions and approaches in outcomes reporting. Health care systems need to keep abreast of these developments as they build their own information infrastructure for outcomes analysis.

Recommended First Steps

Putting in place all of the information support described above is a tall order and, realistically, will take many years. IDNs that work simultaneously on all three fronts—supporting the primary care case manager, ambulatory care sites delivering new care models, and the enterprise overall—will make the quickest progress, provided that each increment is consistent with an eventual integrated solution. On the basis of our research, we believe there are some initial steps that offer immediate value to both efficiency and continuity of care.

Primary care case managers spend much of their time in fragmented tasks relating to patients on their case roster. Basic tools for organizing and recording patient information and tracking follow-up offer immediate efficiencies. These tools can either be provided as stand-alone support or integrated among case managers. The extent to which interfaces provide basic scheduling information (patient and case manager schedules) and basic patient information (care plan, contact information) will determine the efficiency that can be achieved.

For primary care practice sites that are involved in new care models, obvious starting points are the ability to identify and differentiate patients in terms of the assigned care model and care team (in effect, a local registry). Ideally this is integrated with basic displays of patient information that are accessed routinely when patients arrive for care or call for services or information. Another obvious target is capture of the patient care plan. Physicians and case managers interviewed in our research all rated quick access to the care plan—at a minimum from the practice site, but ideally also from home and triage centers—as critical to continuity of care among each patient's designated care team. This is also important for case managers and physicians who provide coverage when the primary team is not available.

At the enterprise level, taking the initial steps toward a patient registry is important. Information such as patient care model, care team members, and routine and emergency procedures and contact information should be available at all telephone and facility access points where patients are likely to present for care or information. With a patient registry in place, it becomes possible even to implement transfers of paper-based information by fax. Obvious initial targets here include quick and reliable communication of hospital discharge summaries and emergency room encounter reports to primary care teams. Another critical element is electronic mail links to facilitate communication among designated caregivers for each patient. The highest priority is probably links among direct care team members.

Conclusions

The information challenges of new models for care management are daunting. Improving information management is critical to accomplishing many of the business objectives for the new process. It will also be a prerequisite to extending the care management principles and process to large numbers of patients and to patient subpopulations beyond those with severe chronic disease.

Realistically, health care systems will make incremental improvements over a long period of time. As they do this, it is important to have a vision of the eventual information infrastructure so that each step is a step in the right direction.

One way to think about requirements and organize the migration path is to work simultaneously at three different levels of the care system: to support the new role of the primary care case manager, improve the operation of the ambulatory care practice site, and address high-priority needs within the enterprise as a whole.

Basic capabilities such as electronic mail connecting providers within the enterprise can offer immediate improvements even before enterprisewide access to patient information can be achieved. For primary care case managers, tools for organizing and remembering patient interactions and coordination tasks can increase both efficiency and effectiveness. Other high priorities are electronic capture of the patients' care plans and information for identifying patients assigned to special care management programs.

Chapter Eight combines the information support discussed in this chapter with an example of a new care model (discussed in Chapter Six) to illustrate how key participants such as a primary care case manager and a primary care physician would interact with information technology as they perform their roles in the new process.

Notes

1. Dick, R. S., Steen, E. B., and Detmer, D. E. (eds.). *The Computer-Based Patient Record: An Essential Technology for Health Care.* Washington, D.C.: National Academy Press, 1997.
2. Schneider, B., and others. *Conceptualizing, Implementing, and Evaluating Extended Care Pathways.* Bloomington, Minn.: National Chronic Care Consortium, 1995.
3. Harris, R. P., O'Malley, M. S., Fletcher, S. W., and Knight, B. P. "Prompting Physicians for Preventive Procedures: A Five-Year Study of Manual and Computer Reminders." *American Journal of Preventive Medicine,* 1990, *6* (3), 145–152.
4. Ware, J. E., and Sherbourne, C. D. "The MOS Thirty-Six-Item Short-Form Health Survey (SF–36)." *Medical Care,* 1992, *30,* 473–483.
5. Eichert, J. H., Wong, H., and Smith, D. R. "The Disease Management Development Process." In W. E. Todd and D. Nash (eds.): *Disease Management: A Systems Approach to Improving Patient Outcomes.* Chicago: American Hospital, 1997.
6. Lush, M. T., Henry, S. B. "Nurses' Use of Health Status Data to Plan for Patient Care: Implications for the Development of a Computer-Based Outcomes Infrastructure." In D. R. Masys (ed.), *1997 AMIA Fall Symposium Conference Proceedings.* Philadelphia: Hanley & Belfus, 1997.
7. Balas, E. A., and others. "Electronic Communication with Patients: Evaluation of Distance Medicine Technology." *Journal of the American Medical Association,* 1997, *278,* 152–159.
8. Ahring, K. K., Ahring, B. P., Joyce, C., and Farid, N. R. "Telephone Modem Access Improves Diabetes Control in Those with Insulin-Requiring Diabetes." *Diabetes Care,* 1992, *15,* 971–975.
9. Friedman, R. H., Stollerman, J. E., Mahoney, D. M., and Rozenblyum, L. "The Virtual Visit: Using Telecommunications Technology to Take Care of Patients." *Journal of the American Medical Informatics Association,* 1997, *4,* 413–425.
10. Osgood-Hynes, D., Ahern, D., Cukor, P., and Penk, W. "Use of an IVR Automated Phone System for Outcome Assessment in a Supported Employment Program for Veterans." Paper presented at the Second Annual Conference of The Information Connection, Emerging Technologies Linking Patients and Providers, Burlington, Vermont, Feb. 1997.
11. Tetzlaff, L. "Consumer Informatics in Chronic Illness." *Journal of the American Medical Informatics Association,* 1997, *4,* 285–300.
12. Flower, J. "Bedside Manna." *Wired,* 1997, *5* (3), 154–155.
13. Wayne-Doppke, J. "Senior Cybersurfers Hit the Net." *Medicine on the Net,* 1997, *3,* 21–25.
14. Eytan, T. "Patient Education: Beyond Handouts." *Medicine on the Net,* 1997, *3,* 24–25.
15. "Intranets Leap the Tower of Babble." *Medicine on the Net,* 1997, *6,* 12.
16. Mullich, J. "Intranet Gives HMO a Shot in the Arm." *PC Week,* 1997, *14,* 27.
17. Chin, T. L. "Patient Education at the Crossroads." *Health Data Management,* 1997, *5,* 106.
18. Brown, E. "Where to Find Medical Advice on the Web." *Fortune,* Mar. 17, 1997, p.162.
19. Jaklevic, M. C. "Internet Technology Moves to Patient-Care Front Lines." *Modern Healthcare,* Mar. 11, 1997, pp. 47–50.
20. Hovey, J. V. "The Potential: Powerful Changes Are Afoot as Health Plans Use Internet Technology for Customer Service." *Healthplan,* 1997, *38,* 41–47.
21. Bell, D. S., and Kahn, C. E. "Health Status Assessment via the Worldwide Web." In *1996 AMIA Annual Fall Symposium.* Philadelphia: Hanley & Belfus, 1996.
22. Kassirer, J. P. "The Next Transformation in the Delivery of Health." *New England Journal of Medicine,* 1995, *322,* 52–54.

23. Jones, M. G. "Telemedicine and the National Information Infrastructure: Are the Realities of Health Care Being Ignored?" *Journal of the American Medical Informatics Association*, 1997, *4*, 399–412.

24. "Touch, But Don't Reach Out." *Modern Healthcare*, 1997, *27*, 40.

25. Sunquist, J. "The Health Village Pilot: Tuning Up an Internet Solution." *Health Management Technology*, 1997, *11*, 38–40.

26. Resultan, E. "Physician Report Cards." *Healthplan*, 1997, *38*, 69–72.

27. Hagland, M. "Ducks in a Row: Experts Offer Practical Advice on Critical Information Systems Strategies for Success in the Emerging World of Quality Report Cards." *Healthplan*, 1997, *38* (2), 23–25.

28. Tarlov, A. R. *National Library of Healthcare Indicators: Health Plan and Network Edition*. Oakbrook Terrace, Ill.: Joint Commission on Accreditation of Healthcare Organizations, 1997.

29. Claus, P. L, and others. "Clinical Care Management and Workflow by Episodes." In D. R. Masys (ed.), *1997 AMIA Fall Symposium Conference Proceedings*. Philadelphia: Hanley & Belfus, 1997.

30. Doyle, J. B. "Health Outcomes: Measuring and Maximizing Value in Disease Management." In W. E. Todd and D. Nash (eds.), *Disease Management: A Systems Approach to Improving Patient Outcomes*. Chicago: American Hospital Publishing, 1997.

CHAPTER EIGHT

CROSS-CONTINUUM CARE MANAGEMENT: A SNAPSHOT OF THE FUTURE PROCESS

Jane Metzger, Derek Messie, and Thomas Hurley

This chapter ties together in a process scenario the new process models described in Chapter Six and the information requirements discussed in Chapter Seven. First-Rate Health System is a fictitious integrated delivery network (IDN) used to illustrate one integrated care model. First-Rate Health includes a medical center, several community hospitals, a medical group of employed primary care and specialist physicians, skilled nursing and rehab services, and home care. It is located in a metropolitan market with several dominant employers that have encouraged employees to select health plans as their health insurance, and the state in which it operates offers Medicare beneficiaries a health plan option. Consequently, 70 percent of First-Rate Health's revenue is prepaid reimbursement. First-Rate Health operates its own health plan, Good Health Plan (GHP), but it also holds contracts with other plans to provide at-risk care.

First-Rate Health has been an integrated system for three years and has evolved considerably from the governance structure and organization of the original individual entities that are now part of First-Rate Health. The first cross-continuum care management process that was piloted and implemented by First-Rate Health targeted elderly patients with chronic diseases. This was the obvious first step, because increasing numbers of patients continue to sign up for Senior Care, GHP's Medicare program.

Under Senior Care, members receive their care in general primary care physician (PCP) practices. First-Rate Health, however, has implemented risk screening as part of its new-member orientation to identify patients who have chronic diseases. Patients are stratified according to their health history and status, and those at greatest risk of deteriorating health are enrolled in the Chronic Care Program. Program participants are assigned to a primary care case manager, who assists the patient's PCP by providing individualized attention. First-Rate Health has also developed wellness and disease management protocols to guide care planning and delivery for patients in the program.

Senior Care and the Chronic Care Program have introduced some new roles into First-Rate Health and enhanced some traditional ones. The changes are illustrated through scenarios for the following roles:

- Primary care case managers coordinate care and provide support and proactive follow-up to patients in the Chronic Care Program. Because First-Rate Health has integrated this role into the primary care team and practice site, case managers participate in clinical assessments and care planning as well.
- PCPs are aided in managing high-risk patients by numerous clinical initiatives, as well as by the primary care case managers. Some care management functions are delegated to primary care case managers. PCPs are kept informed and involved through their own visits with the patients, clinical team meetings, and frequent electronic communications.
- Care management initiatives have added some responsibilities for triage nurses in First-Rate Health's access centers (illustrated in Chapter Five). The additional tasks involve new-member orientation and clinical outreach to patients.
- Patients can take advantage of assistance and tools for self-assessment and personal health management on Web sites maintained by First-Rate Health. The Internet also provides information access to patients and a mode for communicating with care teams at First-Rate Health.

The scenarios in this chapter follow people in each of these roles for a few minutes of a routine day as they participate in First-Rate Health's new care management process.

First-Rate Health has invested heavily in its information technology infrastructure to support the continuum of care with seamless information access and assistance with patient management. The result, the Enterprise System, is the patient care computer system that helps First-Rate Health ensure that there is continuity of care for each patient and that it provides one standard of care and service everywhere in the health system. The scenarios describe how staff use the Enterprise System to accomplish many new tasks and to communicate with one another. The computer desktop for each type of participant is customized to provide easy access to the functions used. The many applications encompassed by the Enterprise System have been integrated so that users move seamlessly from one application to another and the work flows efficiently. Screen shots from this ideal system illustrate system contributions at certain points in the scenarios.

Primary Care Case Manager

Lucinda Bailey is a primary care case manager teamed with two PCPs in the Lockport primary care practice. We join her as she glances at her schedule for the day. She sees that it includes some administrative time to follow up with some of her patients by telephone and catch up on communication and correspondence. She has a few appointments in the clinic, including one with a new patient who will require a case management assessment, and she will make a home visit to one of her patients who has great difficulty coming to the office.

Several urgent messages are flagged on her desktop message counter, and Lucinda opens her in-box to check on these. The first telephone message is from First-Rate Health's access center. A patient, Leonard Barnard, called in the previous night to report problems sleeping (see Figure 8.1). Leonard is enrolled in the Chronic Care Program because of his diabetes, and he was told that someone from his care team would call that day to see how he was doing. Lucinda sets a reminder for herself to call him later in the day, when she has administrative time built into her schedule.

Lucinda's other urgent message concerns Mr. Fiutak, an asthma patient on her case roster who dials into First-Rate Health's intranet every three to four days to download readings from his airway monitor. First-Rate Health has provided Mr. Fiutak with a portable airway monitoring device that records and analyzes peak flow readings and makes treatment recommendations based on the results. The monitor stores readings in its memory and can download via telephone modem into First-Rate Health's Enterprise System, where the results are incorporated into Mr. Fiutak's electronic health record. The Enterprise System also scans the trends in morning and evening readings against the patient's "personal best" value and his normal range of variation. When the rules-based decision support detects a deterioration, the Enterprise System sends an urgent message to Mr. Fiutak's primary care case manager for immediate follow-up.

Lucinda scans the message and clicks to view the flowsheet of recent readings for Mr. Fiutak, as shown in Figure 8.2. As the message suggests, the readings for the last day or so are approaching the red zone on the plot. Lucinda calls the patient immediately and, on the basis of their discussion, decides that Mr. Fiutak should be seen later in the day by the pulmonologist on his team, because he

FIGURE 8.1. ENTERPRISE SYSTEM VIEWED BY PRIMARY CARE CASE MANAGER: PATIENT PHONE NOTE SCREEN.

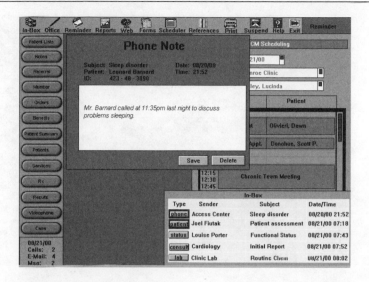

FIGURE 8.2. ENTERPRISE SYSTEM VIEWED BY PRIMARY CARE CASE MANAGER: PATIENT FLOWSHEET SCREEN.

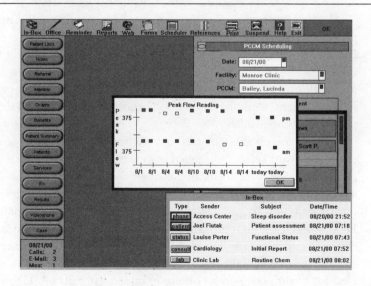

FIGURE 8.3. ENTERPRISE SYSTEM VIEWED BY PRIMARY CARE CASE MANAGER: PATIENT SUMMARY SCREEN.

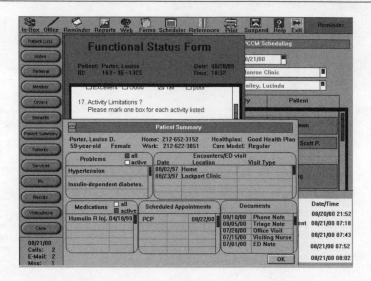

should probably increase his dosage of inhaled steroids. She schedules the appointment and signs the note. A copy, with the flowsheet attached, is transmitted automatically to both Mr. Fiutak's PCP and his pulmonologist.

Lucinda's next message concerns one of her patients, Louise Porter, who has phoned in her weekly functional status assessment using a standard First-Rate Health survey instrument. Patients become quite accustomed to completing the survey by voice response to prerecorded questions. Reporting by telephone is popular with patients because it is free, takes little time, and can be done whenever it is convenient. Compliance with self-reporting has increased since telephone reporting became available.

The Enterprise System uses voice-response technology to convert the answers to the survey into electronic data. Lucinda is notified each time one of her patients completes a self-assessment, because it provides good information on their overall compliance and health status. Self-reporting supplements her own assessments during visits and frequent telephone conversations with her patients. (First-Rate Health also uses the status information in evaluating outcomes to fine-tune the clinical protocols it has developed for the Chronic Care Program.)

Lucinda reviews the results and decides to see when Ms. Porter is next scheduled for a visit. The patient summary screen she calls up (Figure 8.3) shows that Ms. Porter has an appointment in just two days. Lucinda sets a reminder for

FIGURE 8.4. ENTERPRISE SYSTEM VIEWED BY PRIMARY CARE CASE MANAGER: PATIENT RISK STRATIFICATION SCREEN.

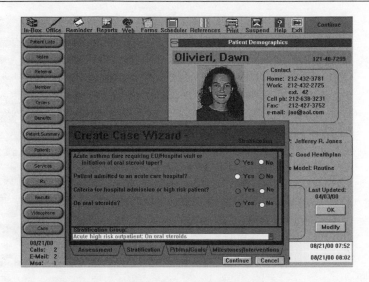

Note: Input on screen content from HBO & Company, based on its Clinical Care Management System.

herself to discuss the survey results with Ms. Porter at that time. This and all other documented patient activities will appear in a patient activity summary (organized by patient) that Lucinda uses for the weekly clinical team meeting.

A reminder comes up on Lucinda's screen. Marjorie Baer's case management plan calls for routine telephone follow-up today. Lucinda decides to call Ms. Baer now. Following their conversation, she writes and signs a brief telephone note in the Enterprise System.

Next Lucinda sees a new patient, Dawn Olivieri, who was treated the previous day in the emergency room. Ms. Olivieri has a long history of asthma and required treatment yesterday because of a particularly bad asthma attack. She was given a nebulizer treatment and put on oral steroids, and an appointment was scheduled with Lucinda to enroll Ms. Olivieri in the Chronic Care Program.

Lucinda greets Ms. Olivieri and signs on to the Enterprise System in the exam room. She identifies Ms. Olivieri in the Enterprise System and then calls up the general asthma history and assessment instrument used by First-Rate Health, which includes the information needed to determine which asthma care model is appropriate. First-Rate Health uses case management software and a case management knowledge base from HBOC. Lucinda requests that the information col-

FIGURE 8.5. ENTERPRISE SYSTEM VIEWED BY PRIMARY CARE CASE MANAGER: PATIENT GOALS/PROBLEMS SCREEN.

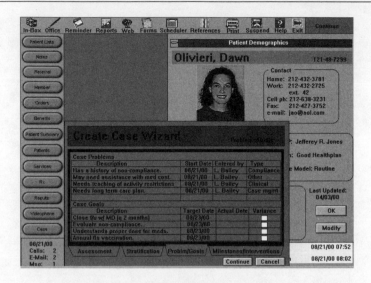

Note: Input on screen content from HBO & Company, based on its Clinical Care Management System.

lected from Ms. Olivieri be analyzed against criteria to determine the appropriate disease management stratification. Based on the information that Lucinda has entered, the system prompts her to ask a few more questions and then suggests a risk stratification, shown in Figure 8.4. As Lucinda suspected, Ms. Olivieri's information places her in the high-risk asthma outpatient stratification. Lucinda indicates her agreement with this classification.

The disease-specific algorithm that appears based on the stratification group determination guides Lucinda during the assessment and subsequent development of a case management plan for Ms. Olivieri. Lucinda administers the screening instrument by asking each question and enters Ms. Olivieri's answers to the questions into the Enterprise System.

Lucinda proceeds to select and set case management goals, as shown in Figure 8.5. The goals displayed have been customized by First-Rate Health to reflect good case management practice for a patient in the acute high-risk asthma outpatient stratification. Lucinda chooses the goals appropriate to Ms. Olivieri and enters the information into the system. After completing this task, she reviews func-

FIGURE 8.6. ENTERPRISE SYSTEM VIEWED BY PRIMARY CARE CASE MANAGER: PATIENT MILESTONES/INTERVENTIONS SCREEN.

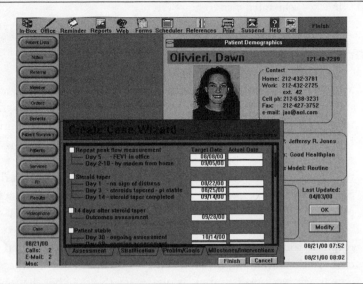

Note: Input on screen content from HBO & Company, based on its Clinical Care Management System.

tional, clinical, and education problems to identify appropriate case management interventions, as shown in Figure 8.6. Lucinda establishes short-term milestones and interventions for the next two weeks, during which Ms. Olivieri will incrementally decrease the dosage of steroids. This will require close monitoring, and Lucinda will contact Ms. Olivieri during this time to see how she is doing.

On the basis of the information entered, the knowledge base in the Enterprise System builds a case management plan for Ms. Olivieri that will guide Lucinda over the next few weeks. Whenever an assessment or an intervention is called for in the plan, Lucinda will receive a prompt and a "to do" item in her case management task list for the day. This will help her ensure that she accomplishes everything in the case management plan, and it will assist First-Rate Health in ensuring that all patients enrolled in the Chronic Care Program receive a single standard of care.

New patients enrolled in the Chronic Care Program receive a complete workup by their clinical team within a few days of intake into the program. Lucinda schedules this visit with Ms. Olivieri's PCP. She also schedules a visit with an asthma education nurse, who will be involved in Ms. Olivieri's care on an ongoing basis. First-Rate Health issues peak flow monitors for self-monitoring to patients in Ms. Olivieri's care model. The asthma education nurses issue the home monitors and coach patients in their use. Once Lucinda has entered the education appointment request, the system assists her in coordinating it with Ms. Olivieri's scheduled visit to her PCP.

Primary Care Physician

We join Dr. Subeeka Reedy at the beginning of her clinic session. She has a few minutes to review her schedule and catch up on the messages that arrived in her in-box overnight. She will spend most of her time in the clinic today but also has a scheduled meeting of the clinical practice committee, which develops and maintains protocols for clinical practice initiatives of First-Rate Health. Initially this group targeted care management of patients enrolled in the Chronic Care Support Program; now, however, they are beginning to roll out care management protocols and clinical outreach to broader patient populations.

Subeeka's in-box contains a mixture of communications: consult and laboratory reports for her patients and messages from the extended care team in her clinic and elsewhere in the care system. She opens the first message (Figure 8.7), which was sent by a community pharmacy to notify her that one of her patients is a week late for a refill for a blood pressure control medication.

FIGURE 8.7. ENTERPRISE SYSTEM VIEWED BY PRIMARY CARE PHYSICIAN: COMMUNITY PHARMACY MESSAGE SCREEN.

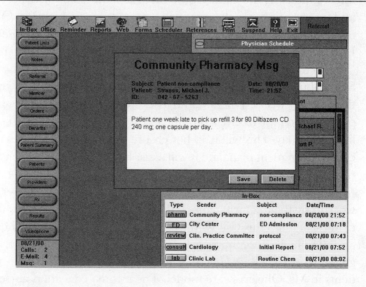

GHP's prescription benefit allows patients to patronize a number of community pharmacies. Because these pharmacies are linked electronically, prescriptions can be transmitted to the location each patient prefers. This allows pharmacies not only to have medications prepared before patients arrive to pick them up but also to notify PCPs when a patient fails to pick up a prescription or refill. Because it has been able to track prescriptions in this way, First-Rate Health has found significant noncompliance, especially with chronic medications. The clinical practice committee has set aggressive targets for increasing compliance. One approach is this automatic notification when patients fail to pick up prescribed medications or refills, but they are also piloting new types of patient education and counseling to address noncompliance.

The patient in question, Michael Strauss, is now a week overdue in picking up the blood pressure medication. Subeeka decides that she will call the patient to assess the situation and reinforce the importance of complying with the treatment plan; she sets a reminder for herself to do so later in the day, during the time set aside for her administrative tasks. During the conversation she will encourage Mr. Strauss to participate in a telephone hypertension program, in which a nurse education specialist provides coaching and information in weekly group discussions and is also available for individual counseling. So far, patients have been happy with the program, and initial results indicate that the compliance of participating patients may be improving. Mr. Strauss seems a good candidate for the program because he has been noncompliant in the past and has other identified risk factors for coronary artery disease. Subeeka completes and signs a referral request to the nurse who runs the program; an information packet and enrollment form will automatically be sent to the patient.

The next message informs Subeeka that one of her patients enrolled in the Chronic Care Support Program was seen the previous night in the emergency room. The Enterprise System automatically notifies the patient's PCP and primary care case manager of unplanned interventions. Subeeka sends a message to her case manager requesting that she follow up with Edward Slater by telephone and get an update from the visiting nurse who is due to visit the patient today in his home.

The third message is a reminder from the chairman of the clinical practice committee about today's meeting and advance copies of the protocols they will review (see Figure 8.8). One agenda item is recommended changes to one of the dosing algorithms used in the clinical protocol for patients with congestive heart failure; another is a proposed revision to patient education materials for patients with newly diagnosed asthma. Subeeka prints these out so she can review them in advance of the meeting.

FIGURE 8.8. ENTERPRISE SYSTEM VIEWED BY PRIMARY CARE PHYSICIAN: PRINTOUT OF PROTOCOLS FOR REVIEW.

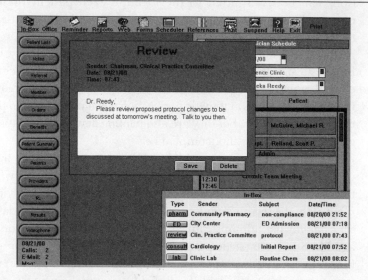

Triage Nurse in Access Center

The access center is involved in the Chronic Care Support Program and clinical outreach to First-Rate Health patients in several ways. To illustrate, we join Adelle Wilder, the triage nurse in the access center, as she spends part of her day on related tasks.

Triage nurses are assigned to take incoming calls or perform call-outs according to a personal schedule displayed on their PCs. Supervisors alter schedules and assignments throughout the day as needed to ensure that First-Rate Health's service standards are always met. During slow call periods, triage nurses have scheduled time to perform outreach.

Adelle clicks Outreach on her computer workstation and reviews a work list of patient contacts. The first call is to William Alexander, a new enrollee in Senior Care. First-Rate Health arranges a welcome telephone call to explain Senior Care's approach to providing care for senior citizens, to ensure that Mr. Alexander has designated a PCP, and to administer a risk-screening survey to identify whether he can benefit from the Chronic Care Support Program.

After reaching Mr. Alexander by telephone, Adelle administers the risk-screening survey, shown in Figure 8.9. She records Mr. Alexander's answers in the Enterprise System, which analyzes the results immediately to produce a score. Based on

FIGURE 8.9. ENTERPRISE SYSTEM VIEWED BY TRIAGE NURSE: NEW-MEMBER RISK SCREENING SCREEN.

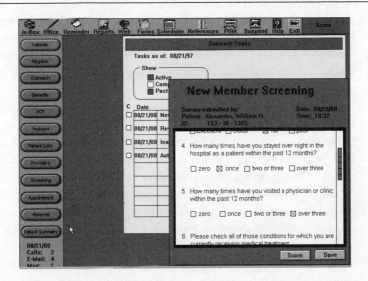

the score for this patient, the system prompts her to enroll him in the Chronic Care Support Program. Adelle explains how the program works and, with Mr. Alexander's agreement, enrolls him in the program. (This changes his care model assignment from "routine" to "Chronic Care Program" in the patient registry maintained in the Enterprise System.)

Mr. Alexander selected Dr. Martin as his PCP when he enrolled, so Adelle schedules a home assessment visit by Dr. Martin's primary care case manager. Scheduled as soon as possible after enrollment in the Chronic Care Program, these visits allow case managers to assess both patient status and the home environment to identify medical and environmental problems that require immediate attention. Initial home visits are followed by a complete workup in the clinic, involving the patient's PCP, case manager, and appropriate specialist physicians. As Adelle arranges to fax orientation materials to Mr. Alexander, she muses about the increasing number of senior citizens who are equipped with fax machines and who are adept browsers on the Internet!

Her next call-out is to another new member of Senior Care, who completed and submitted the risk-screening instrument on GHP's Web site. Scoring for this patient indicates that she can be assigned to the regular care of a PCP (what First-Rate Health calls the routine care model). Adelle reaches Kara Marshall by telephone, welcomes her to Senior Care, and assists her in selecting an appropriate PCP in a clinic near her home. She enters the selection criteria and describes the PCP candidate who has been selected by the system because he meets Ms. Marshall's criteria and is currently accepting new patients. Ms. Marshall agrees to sign on with Dr. Donaldson. Adelle notes this in the system and schedules an initial visit in the next month. She explains the Senior Care program and describes how Ms. Marshall can obtain services and information. She also requests an automatic mail-out of a complete orientation packet to Ms. Marshall's home. This will include information about a number of senior wellness programs and a welcome letter from Dr. Donaldson.

Adelle opens her next outreach task notice, which is for an inactive patient. The Enterprise System flags Senior Care patients for follow-up when no encounters or telephone interactions have occurred for six months. Adelle reaches the patient, Betty von Bulow, who tells her that she has enrolled with another health plan (apparently the membership update has not yet reached the Enterprise System). Adelle records the change in enrollment status, which automatically triggers the preparation and mail-out of a letter to the patient, accompanied by a patient satisfaction survey, as shown in Figure 8.10. First-Rate Health monitors patient satisfaction very closely and tracks patients' reasons for disenrollment to identify aspects of care and customer service that should be targeted for improvement. Because of the importance of obtaining feedback from patients who disenroll, each survey sent out is tracked. If it is not returned within three weeks, the patient is contacted by telephone to administer the survey.

FIGURE 8.10. ENTERPRISE SYSTEM VIEWED BY TRIAGE NURSE: DISENROLLMENT SURVEY DELIVERY SCREEN.

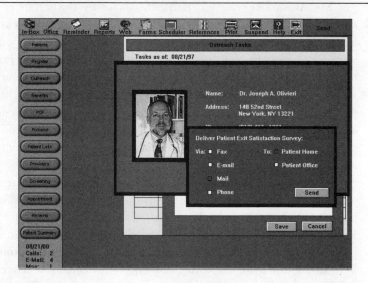

Each week the Enterprise System scans encounters, claims, and clinical information to identify patients who are potential candidates for the Chronic Care Support Program. This is one mechanism that First-Rate Health uses to identify patients with recently diagnosed chronic illness or service utilization that suggests deteriorating health status. Identified patients are assigned to a triage nurse for follow-up.

The next call in Adelle's outreach work list is to a patient identified by this scan of the database. The patient, Pamela Metzger, has had two recent urgent care encounters and one emergency room visit, which tripped the total-cost-of-care trigger in the rules used to screen the database. Ms. Metzger has a history of asthma, but the severity and frequency of her problems clearly have worsened.

Adelle sends a message to the PCP, as shown in Figure 8.11, asking him to review the patient's recent health history to see if he agrees that Ms. Metzger should be enrolled in the Chronic Care Support Program. If the PCP agrees, Adelle will call Ms. Metzger, offer enrollment, provide orientation information, and schedule an assessment visit with the PCP and other care team members as soon as possible.

Patient

Louise Porter is a Senior Care patient enrolled in the Chronic Care Support Program. A retired computer company executive, she is one grandmother who does

FIGURE 8.11. ENTERPRISE SYSTEM VIEWED BY TRIAGE NURSE: PCP REMINDER SCREEN.

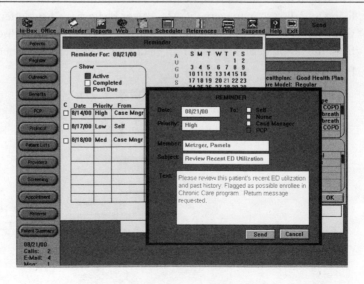

not need her grandchildren to show her how to access the Internet. She has a PC in her study at home and uses it frequently to communicate with her care team at First-Rate Health, as well as to obtain information and services.

Ms. Porter accesses the GHP Web site and enters her ID code and password to reach the restricted area for Senior Care patients. A message posted for Louise by the rules-based decision support in the Enterprise System reminds her that it is time to complete a functional status survey, as she does each month.

First-Rate Health tries to obtain functional status updates on a regular basis from patients in the Chronic Care Support Program; some patients prefer to use the telephone option, but Ms. Porter usually enters hers on the Web site. She answers the questions and submits her self-assessment. This is automatically scored, and the results are routed to her PCP and primary care case manager. When the results are worse than a patient's baseline functional status, the rules-based decision alerts the care team immediately.

Next, Ms. Porter accesses a message function on the Web site. Her visiting nurse, Jane Richards, is due to arrive at Ms. Porter's home the next morning. The doorbell is out of order, so Ms. Porter leaves a message for Ms. Richards to call ahead on her car telephone rather than rely on the doorbell. Ms. Richards is connected to the Enterprise System via a laptop computer, and she dials in periodically to download documentation and pick up changes in her schedule and communications from patients, the home care office, and First-Rate Health providers involved in the care of her patients.

Ms. Porter has diabetes and belongs to a patient support group organized by GHP. The group chats regularly on-line, has educational group chats, puts out a newsletter, and shares recipes and other suggestions relating to activities of daily living and disease management. Ms. Porter reviews the newsletter and is reminded that one of her chat group friends, Elizabeth Rowden, was discharged recently from the hospital. She sends her an electronic note welcoming her back to the support group.

CHAPTER NINE

BEST PRACTICES IN ENTERPRISE INFORMATION MANAGEMENT FOR INTEGRATED DELIVERY NETWORKS

Peter Kilbridge and Erica Drazen

The past decade has seen a frenzy of merger activity among provider institutions to form large integrated delivery networks (IDNs). Because these organizations are for the most part young and still very much in the process of integrating (as discussed earlier in this book), there is limited understanding of how best to manage the unique information systems challenges facing such large, disparate organizations.

To learn more about how leading IDNs are approaching these challenges, we performed a study of information management practices at ten prominent IDNs.[1] In the initial study we identified some emerging practice themes. We continue to follow these themes both with the original study organizations and through other fieldwork. This chapter integrates information from all these sources.

The original study sites were selected from a list of candidates judged by our experts to be demonstrating innovative approaches to information systems management, business process integration, or both. The study sites are as follows:

HealthSystem Minnesota	Minneapolis, Minnesota
Henry Ford Health System	Detroit, Michigan
Integris Health	Oklahoma City, Oklahoma
Intermountain Health Care	Salt Lake City, Utah

North Mississippi Health Services   Tupelo, Mississippi

Partners HealthCare System   Boston, Massachusetts

ProMedica Health System   Toledo, Ohio

Providence Health Systems   Portland, Oregon

Sentara Health System   Norfolk, Virginia

University Medical Center, Tucson   Tucson, Arizona

Our researchers launched the study by conducting site visits and interviewing information systems (IS) management, executive management, and clinician users to ask the following questions:

Is the CIO involved in organizationwide strategic planning? If so, how?

What is your process for IS strategic planning?

How do your organization's executive and IS management assess the value of IS investments?

What is the organizational structure of your IS department?

How is your IS governed?

How do you manage the challenges of implementing advanced technologies?

What role has the IS department played during organizational mergers?

What is the role of clinical staff in your IS organization?

In interpreting the information gathered from assembled background materials and interviews, we faced a serious dilemma. We had selected IDNs that we believed would illustrate advanced practices in various aspects of IS management. How would we now determine whether a given practice was successful, or more generally, what makes a practice "advanced"? To address this question we examined several indicators of organizational function.

We sought evidence that a practice supports the execution of some element or elements of organizational strategy. An initiative whose stated and demonstrated objective is, for example, to facilitate availability of patient information across care settings clearly supports an organizational strategic goal of integrating cross-continuum care processes. A difficulty arose here because some of the organizations studied were in the early stages of organizational integration, making it premature at the time of the site visits to evaluate the success of some initiatives. In these cases we looked for appropriate alignment of practices and strategic objectives and tried to assess the likelihood of success, given the organization's structure, function, and resources. We also attempted to develop an impression of how well each IS department functioned overall:

> How closely aligned were the philosophies of the CIO and other IDN executives?
>
> How closely did the CIO's assessment of the organization's function match our observations from discussions with division and line managers and users?
>
> Were strategic initiatives going forward according to plan and within budget?

All of these criteria are, of course, subjective measures, based largely on the observations of the interviewers. Nonetheless, we felt at the conclusion of each site visit that we had succeeded in assembling an accurate and coherent impression of each organization. Our observations and impressions were supported by our prior and subsequent experience at these sites. Appendix B contains comparative information on the size and degree of integration that characterize the study organizations.

At the conclusion of the study, we sponsored a one-day forum for the participating CIOs for the purpose of discussing the findings. The forum was attended by representatives of seven of the ten organizations, and the meeting yielded some valuable additional insights that have been incorporated into this chapter.

When information from the ten sites was synthesized, a number of themes became apparent that suggest some best practices and key success factors for IS management in IDNs. These themes are illustrated in Figure 9.1 and discussed in detail in this chapter.

Executive Commitment to the Strategic Importance of Information Systems

The Importance of Executive Commitment

> *Best practices:* Ongoing efforts to gain commitment of an organization's executive management to information systems as a strategic asset are essential to the successful function of an IS department. CIOs must work to develop and reinforce executive commitment through educational efforts with executive management.

Clear commitment of the executive management team to information systems as a strategic asset is crucial to the success of the organization's IS department. Such commitment is necessary to promote consistent, long-term investment in strategic IS projects and to permit proper control over IS management and standards.

FIGURE 9.1. TEN RULES FOR INFRASTRUCTURE MANAGEMENT.

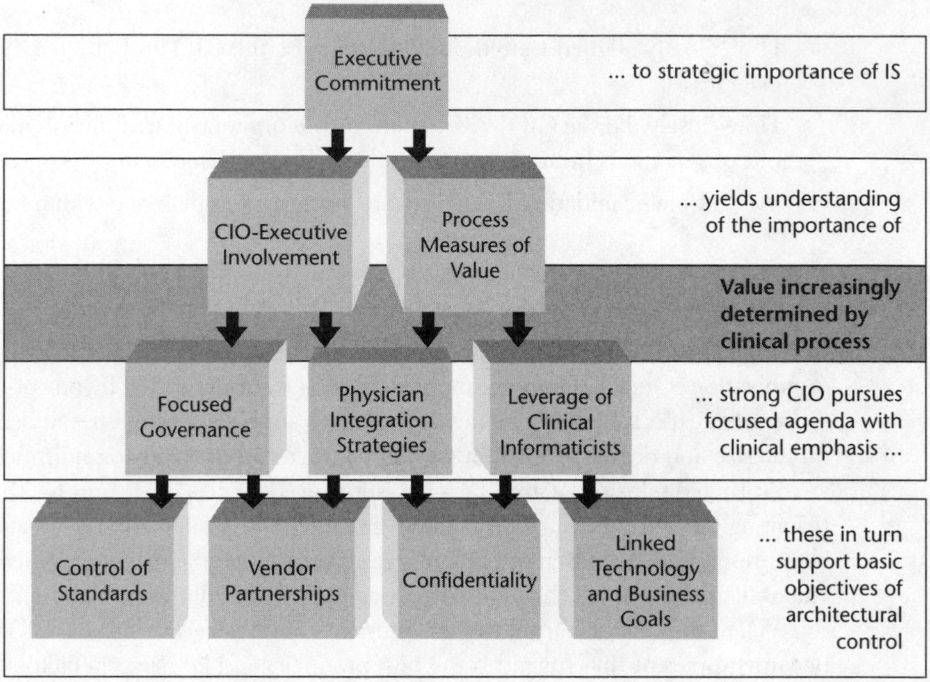

Executive Commitment

... to strategic importance of IS

CIO-Executive Involvement

Process Measures of Value

... yields understanding of the importance of

Value increasingly determined by clinical process

Focused Governance

Physician Integration Strategies

Leverage of Clinical Informaticists

... strong CIO pursues focused agenda with clinical emphasis ...

Control of Standards

Vendor Partnerships

Confidentiality

Linked Technology and Business Goals

... these in turn support basic objectives of architectural control

Copyright © 1998 by First Consulting Group.

Organizations that demonstrated executive-level commitment to information systems did so in several ways. They made substantial and long-term (three- to five-year) capital budget commitments for information technology investments. Our study participants dedicated an average of 26 percent of their capital budgets to information systems, compared with the 1997 College of Healthcare Information Management Executives survey's average of 19 percent[2] (see Appendix B). In general, a higher priority was placed on investments in technology for enterprise connectivity and information integration than on end-user application development, at least until the former was well established. Strategic business planning incorporated IS initiatives, and perhaps most important, the CIO routinely participated in strategic business planning.

CIOs face constant demands from a myriad of constituencies for new applications, new functionality in old applications, and more or better service. At the same time, the CIO must address a set of IDN infrastructure demands of which most users are unaware, such as enterprisewide patient identification, connectivity, and the establishment of a clinical data repository. The CIO requires strong executive support for investment in these unglamorous yet vital enterprise system integration projects in order to apply the necessary resources successfully.

One recently formed IDN identified early on the strategic importance of investment in such systems for integration and specifically recruited a new CIO who shared this vision. Reporting directly to the CEO and an accepted member of the executive group, the CIO successfully installed a robust enterprise network infrastructure and inaugurated a new clinical data repository in less than eighteen months.

One of the oldest IDNs in our study established an approach to the patient identification challenge based on enterprise registration more than a decade ago. Inclusion of IS investment as a specific priority of its business plan over the years has resulted in the development of one of the most smoothly functioning enterprise information systems we have observed, with multiple rural hospitals connected by a high-speed wide-area network and a common user interface across all major settings.

In IDNs where executive support for information systems was less clear, we observed a variety of problems. Communication between the executive team and the CIO was shaky, and the CIOs were frequently frustrated in their efforts to interpret executive direction and commitment to IS projects. One of these organizations also exhibited somewhat schizophrenic approaches to strategic investments, with a requirement for strict return on investment (ROI) justification for all projects, including strategic investments. Another CIO contemplated resorting to "charge-back" arrangements to control user demands for services, whereas the chief financial officer (CFO) at the same organization described the charge-back concept as "funny money" and counterproductive to organizational objectives. This CIO was receiving inconsistent messages and support from the executive team.

Cultivating Executive Commitment to Information Systems

CIOs must strive continually to educate occupants of the executive suite on the importance of information systems to the organization's strategic goals. Many of the CIOs who participated in the study remarked that the cultivation of executive and board-level commitment to information systems is a never-ending task. In executing this ongoing educational role, the CIO should take advantage of every opportunity for visibility before the CEO, other senior executives, and members of the board to explain and remind them of the objectives and strategic reasoning behind ongoing, high-cost strategic investments in particular.

Several study participants emphasized the importance of the physician role in gaining executive support. "Physicians are highly influential with the executive team, and we underutilize them," said one CIO. Another described his organization's use of physician-executive teams for major IS initiatives, which ensures close collaboration between these groups and reinforces their commitment to the successful execution of projects.

One CIO felt that one of the functions most valued by the executive team at his institution is that of interpreter between the IS department and executives—the use of his ability to simplify information technology concepts for executive consumption. Other participants agreed that such communication skills are particularly valued by executives because they are relatively scarce among technical personnel. Properly leveraging this interpreter role is central to the ongoing cultivation of executive commitment to information systems.

The CIO forum participants discussed the challenge of gaining support from executives, board members, and ultimately users for IS investments. Participants emphasized first and foremost that it is essential for CIOs to have an intimate understanding of the "sales process" at their institutions. Such an understanding has multiple aspects. The CIO must be able to identify the key constituents—executives, board members, and physicians—whose buy-in is critical to investing in IS initiatives. In addition, the CIO must be sensitive both to the proper approach to enlisting support, given the organization's unique cultural considerations, and to the particular priorities and personal styles of each key constituent. The successful sales process thus involves presenting initiatives through the appropriate political and cultural channels while simultaneously developing a customized presentation for each target audience. Pilot programs that address the specific needs of key constituents may be needed to sell an overall package.

Another aspect of cultivating support for investments involves establishing an ongoing background public relations effort aimed at publicizing IS achievements, particularly relating to customer service and the department's ability to deliver on user requests. One organization publishes a regular IS newsletter. Another sets aggressive service goals and has publicized its success in achieving some of these—for example, resolution of 80 percent of customer questions in less than ten minutes.

Forum participants also agreed that sales efforts directed at executives and board members must focus on the information system's ability to solve business problems, not technology problems. As a corollary, it is essential that business sponsors and executives take some ownership for the success or failure of IS initiatives. When they do, the organization is more likely to work through implementation challenges successfully, and it improves the IS department's credibility with executives over time, thereby making the sales task easier in the future.

Building a Foundation of Understanding

CIO Involvement in Enterprise Strategic Planning

Although most health care executives acknowledge the importance of information systems to the IDN's business objectives, a true understanding of the value of information as a strategic asset that merits executive-level involvement and substantial investment is less common. Increasingly, enlightened executives realize that the information systems function within their organizations deserves a presence in the executive suite. For example, effective organizational strategic planning for the IDN can no longer be carried out in the absence of the CIO. IS representation is vital to permit proactive planning for evolving enterprise information requirements and to manage executive expectations of information systems regarding budgetary and time implications of new initiatives, such as purchasing a large physician practice or another hospital. The specific reporting relationship (whether the CIO reports to the CEO, for example) is not critical, as long as the CIO participates in crucial discussions that affect enterprise strategy.

Several CIO forum participants noted that the importance of a direct reporting relationship to the CEO may vary within an organization over time. Direct reporting may be necessary at the outset to demonstrate the CIO's mandate, but in the long run it is more important that the reporting relationship be with an engaged executive, whether or not it is the CEO. One participant further emphasized this point, citing the distinction between "ego and effectiveness"—the importance of reporting to an engaged executive, regardless of title, rather than insisting on reporting to the CEO.

The practical limits of CIO involvement in organizational strategic planning were cited by several participants. One noted that although CIOs must be in touch with strategic thinking, they do not have the time to be involved in every business decision. Strong communication links with other executives are important here, to help the CIO track important strategic issues that are "on the radar screen" in the event that they should begin to require IS involvement.

How Do You Measure Value?

Best practices: The value of strategic initiatives should be subject to a justification process that considers both likely contributions to organizational strategic goals and evidence of value demonstrated in other organizations. The traditional ROI analyses should be broadened to include a focus on noneconomic returns on investment or returns that are difficult to express in dollar terms.

Assessing the value contributed by information systems was one of the topics of greatest interest to our participants, and our study revealed some interesting philosophies regarding how—or whether—to "measure" value.

At leading IDNs, the era of traditional ROI analysis of investments in strategic information systems is past. Executives at most of the participating IDNs evaluate these investments according to their perception of the system's contribution to the business processes it supports. In the case of basic IS infrastructure investments—network infrastructure, enterprisewide patient identification, and clinical data repository—these processes are considered the equivalent of bricks and mortar, that is, essential to doing business as an IDN. In one IDN that persisted with a requirement for ROI justification of strategic projects, we observed a fragmented and inconsistent approach to investment in and implementation of its clinical data repository and enterprisewide patient identification initiatives.

Furthermore, executives in advanced IDNs increasingly recognize the importance of enterprise clinical processes among the organization's core business processes. The delivery of high-quality, cross-continuum care and the ability to demonstrate quality and efficiency to payers are becoming threshold competencies for IDNs in the era of managed care. Accordingly, the executives we interviewed sought improvements in process and outcomes measures of care to demonstrate the value of investments in information systems: reduced length of inpatient stay, improved adherence to clinical guidelines and uniform standards of care across the enterprise, and better leverage in managed care contracting, resulting from easy access to data, that demonstrates reduced costs and improved outcomes.

One CIO emphasized the importance of proxy measures of the value of information systems—the most important of which is the question, "Do people use the system?" As obvious as this seems, the industry is replete with examples of systems that are underutilized because of some combination of faulty planning, design, user education, marketing, implementation, and support.

Another aspect of new approaches to analyzing the value of systems is reflected in the willingness of study participants to justify their strategic initiatives on the basis of published experience from the industry. One study organization used cost figures from published studies to estimate the savings to be gained by introducing rules-based decision support into its enterprise clinical information systems.

The trend away from traditional ROI analysis and toward consideration of strategic contribution and information technology–enabled process outcomes is echoed in industries outside of health care. CIOs in the manufacturing world increasingly view information technology investments as supportive of business objectives and core processes, such as improving customer satisfaction or optimizing workflow.[3,4] In a recent interview, the CIO of Fidelity Investments likened the process for justifying information technology investments to the research and development function in pharmaceutical companies. Rather than seeking an immediate ROI, Fidelity invests heavily in information technology, with the expectation that the investments will take years to justify themselves.[5]

There is evidence that the health care industry is moving in the same direction. In a survey conducted by the Computer-Based Patient Records Institute, CIOs report that when considering computer-based patient records systems, the assessment approach they most commonly use for strategic investments is to assess the quantitative and qualitative benefits of the system (58 percent), followed by cost analysis (49 percent) and prediction of improvement in key performance indicators (34 percent). Only one-third of the respondents reported that they performed a formal cost-benefit analysis, and one-tenth performed no formal assessment of value at all. Infrastructure investments, on the other hand, are likely to be evaluated on the basis of cost (63 percent).[6]

There remains an interest in developing better methods for postimplementation evaluation of systems investments than currently exist. Although some academic organizations have informatics research groups whose tasks include analyzing systems performance and impact on clinical practice, most IS departments do not have such resources. Measures of system utilization and of user satisfaction and productivity may help to address this need.

Pursuit of a Focused Agenda

Information Systems Governance

> *Best practices:* (1) Benchmark organizations tend to concentrate effective governance among small groups of senior management (sometimes almost entirely with the CIO, which is not a model for everyone). (2) New organizational structures can confront the difficulties of cross-continuum care delivery and thereby address one of the most challenging aspects of IDN function.

Governance means simply the structures and individuals responsible for decision making. Among our study organizations, the nature of the governance of the IS department is changing. Most of the leading IDNs have deemphasized the role of the IS steering committee, in some cases eliminating it altogether. Decision making is increasingly concentrated in the hands of small groups of executives. At one extreme, one organization in the study places essentially full responsibility for IS governance—strategic planning, budgetary decisions, and high-level-priority setting—in the hands of its CIO. Another uses an IS steering committee that is essentially controlled by the CFO, who oversees the IS department.

Although key decisions for information systems, especially decisions on project prioritization and budgeting, are being made by fewer individuals, highly functioning IDNs have mechanisms in place to ensure that needs and strategy are adequately communicated across all levels of the organization. In large organizations, local entity representation of IS may be necessary to ensure proper attention to diverse constituent needs and to implement systems effectively at the local level. Organizational structures for information systems are discussed shortly.

Involvement of users in systems development and implementation is another essential element of the communications process. One study organization redesigned its systems implementation approach to incorporate end-user input during system design, selection, and development, with the goal of achieving user consensus on major IS initiatives prior to proceeding with implementation. The buy-in achieved in this manner allows the IS department to subsequently follow a regimented implementation schedule—without the need for extensive user negotiations along the way.

An interesting hypothesis offered by several participants involves the importance of strong central governance of IS as an IDN evolves. They suggested that in the early stages of IDN consolidation a strong central IS authority is essential in order to drive standards across the organization; it may subsequently become less important, and greater flexibility to accommodate local needs may become feasible and desirable.

Organizational Structures for Information Systems Departments

Best practices: The IS organizational structure should mirror overall organizational processes, which should in turn support integration across an organization's functional, clinical, and geographical settings.

Organizational structures of information systems for IDNs have evolved from those of acute-care hospitals, and in smaller organizations they may be indistinguishable from a traditional hospital structure. In the simplest case, IS divisions represent major enterprisewide functions: network and telecommunications, financial systems, operations, clinical applications, and so on. In contrast with the single-hospital setting, however, the IDN structure must incorporate enterprise integration functions such as enterprisewide patient identification, a clinical data repository, and applications interface groups (see Figure 9.2).

Most larger IDNs incorporate another dimension into the IS organizational structure: local entity representation. The result is a matrix organization, with staff jointly responsible to a local individual (such as a hospital IS director) and an enterprise director (a director of network services, for example) (see Figure 9.3). Such a two-dimensional approach to organizational structure appears to be unavoidable in large IDNs, given the need to provide adequate flexibility to address the unique needs of different environments. This is particularly true given the historical evolution of most IDNs, in which previously unaffiliated institutions with different financial, clinical, and administrative processes and cultures have recently merged.

The challenge of working in matrix organizations was the central theme in our discussion of organization at the CIO forum. One participant stated that complexity of organizational structures "is getting weirder all the time and will continue to get weirder" as IDNs develop matrices within matrices to address the combination of cross-setting and setting-specific needs and, increasingly, the development of information systems–supported "virtual networks" with external organizations. Participants agreed that the great challenge posed by the matrix organization is the conflict between improved flexibility for service provision

FIGURE 9.2. ONE-DIMENSIONAL ORGANIZATIONAL STRUCTURE: FUNCTIONAL.

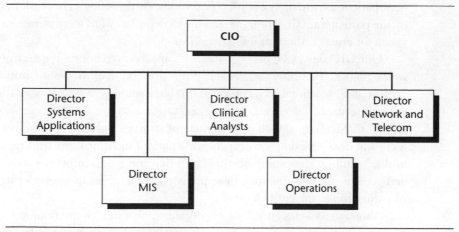

FIGURE 9.3. TWO-DIMENSIONAL ORGANIZATIONAL STRUCTURE: GEOGRAPHICAL AND FUNCTIONAL.

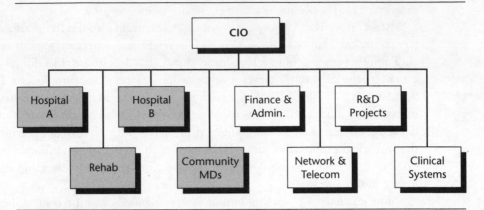

across the IDN and decreased accountability resulting from multiple reporting relationships.

One participating organization took an additional step toward addressing the need to provide continuity of information across the enterprise in support of evolving cross-continuum patient care. This IDN created a division of IS responsible specifically for the "care continuum" (Figure 9.4). The director of this division is responsible for tracking patient flow across the enterprise and coordinating the participating elements of information systems to ensure the availability of relevant patient information in different settings. At the study's conclusion, another of the participant CIOs reorganized his IS department to incorporate such a division for cross-continuum information support.

One CIO described his organization's approach to improving accountability in the matrix. The IDN assigns account representatives to specific initiatives to achieve staff accountability. Although this has been successful, he pays additional costs in terms of overhead. This organization also has an "enterprise systems group" that is charged with management of strategic enterprise initiatives such as a clinical data repository, enterprisewide patient identification, and registration and scheduling. His experience has been that the group improves coordination across entities in implementing these projects but has difficulty engendering a sense of ownership at the entity level.

Although well-designed business organizational models are reinforced by parallel IS department organizational structure, the converse is also true. One organization had semi-independent business-line "silos" that did not support

FIGURE 9.4. TWO-DIMENSIONAL ORGANIZATIONAL STRUCTURE: FUNCTIONAL AND PROCESS.

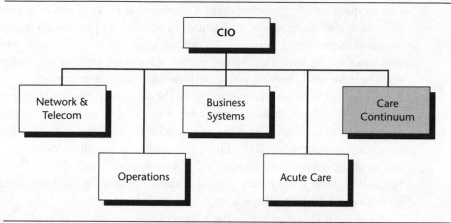

Copyright © 1998 by First Consulting Group.

development of cross-continuum enterprise processes, and the construction of a parallel information system did not help—it supported intraenterprise competition, severely impeding the development of infrastructure for integration.

The Role of Information Systems in Promoting Integration Strategies

Mergers: The Role of the Information Systems Department

Best practices: CIOs must be involved from the outset in planning for organizational change in order to be able to position information systems to facilitate integration processes.

Mergers are a frequent occurrence among today's provider organizations, and IS departments are often expected to play a crucial role, providing the infrastructure that pulls the organization together. At the same time, CIOs all too frequently find themselves involved in the process as an afterthought. As a result, they may be caught in the middle of the political turmoil surrounding the merger, unable to facilitate the process proactively. One of our CIOs told of the difficulties encountered when he was left out of crucial budget meetings surrounding a merger (the organization neglected to consider one hospital's budget for software maintenance). If the IS department is to assist with operational integration during the merger, the CIO must be part of the planning process from its outset.

CIOs agreed on several principles for handling the human resources aspects of organizational mergers. First, one is better off making staff consolidation decisions quickly and executing them with minimal delay. The CIOs agreed that they were able to determine quite quickly who would perform in the new environment. A prolonged consolidation process is not necessarily viewed as more fair; moreover, it may have the result of encouraging your stronger employees to look elsewhere for work, leaving you with those who have fewer options.

Second, it is important to appreciate the amount of stress placed on staff by a merger. Workloads shift, often unpredictably, as staff consolidate; stronger staff members may find themselves bearing an increased burden of responsibility, with no apparent benefit to them. This can rapidly lead to demoralization. Proper preparation, ongoing assessment and acknowledgment of your staff's extraordinary efforts, and if necessary, getting outside assistance to help people make the transition can be highly beneficial.

The need for attending to the effects of the merger on IS staff was a recurring theme among CIO forum participants. Several CIOs pointed out that this is particularly important in an industry where salaries are generally lower than in the market at large; indeed, all participants voiced frustration with the difficulty of getting and keeping good people, and several cited problems with staff morale during the merger process. At the same time, one participant observed that one will likely lose good people who cannot adjust to new environmental realities—and that such people should be encouraged to go, as they will otherwise pose an impediment to integration.

There were two schools of thought among participants regarding the value of the early merging of IS departments. Several CIOs felt that mergers offer an extraordinary opportunity for IS to lead the organization and that early consolidation can produce large, immediate gains. Other participants felt that organizations should merge IS functions "only when the reasons are clearly compelling" in terms of the predictable, short-term gains that will be demonstrated. These differing views stem from the fact that the merger process for IS constitutes a five- to seven-year cycle and produces an immediate two-year decrease in efficiency.

Several people emphasized the importance of cultivating the organization's "opinion leaders" in favor of the merger. Given an awareness of the magnitude of change anticipated, such individuals can be invaluable champions of the merger process during difficult times.

Information Systems Support for Physician Integration

Best practices: (1) IDNs must identify the importance of integrating physicians into enterprise clinical and business processes, and they must leverage information systems to support these integration efforts. (2) Providing electronic access to basic clinical data for physicians across the enterprise must be a high-priority goal for the IS department. Innovative approaches should be considered to provide this access as quickly as possible. (3) Information systems should support specific processes of physician integration—especially disease management and referral management—as these processes are redesigned across the enterprise.

The business demands of managed care are altering the alignment of incentives and creating a new level of interdependence between IDNs and their affiliated physicians. Two major environmental forces are driving this new alignment of incentives: increased financial risk sharing between IDNs and physicians, and competition among IDNs for physicians.

Risk bearing provides financial incentives to manage the practice of medicine so as to maximize the efficiency and quality of care provision and to document the resulting improvements in quality and cost savings. IDNs and physicians sharing risk through capitated contracts are therefore implementing aggressive programs for disease management: management of the care of members/patients across the continuum of care, according to the principles of evidence-based medicine. Internal management of referrals according to medical necessity, rather than strictly according to payer rules, also becomes increasingly important. Competition among IDNs for physicians provides further incentive to organizations to make it easier and more appealing for physicians to work with the IDN—by providing easy access to hospital data and by streamlining cumbersome processes such as referral management.

Approaches to Information Systems Support for Disease Management. Proper disease management is dependent on IS support at several levels:

- Providers need access to basic clinical data for any member, from all settings across the enterprise.
- Point-of-care use of information systems by physicians will improve the quality of clinical data capture and allow real-time decision support for patient care.
- An enterprise data management strategy and data model will permit the storage and analysis of these data from settings across the IDN, providing the data management necessary for real-time clinical decision support and enabling retrospective analysis of aggregate data for assessment of utilization, practice patterns, and outcomes of care.

Providing Access to Patient Clinical Data from Across the Enterprise—Today. We have observed two general approaches to provision of information from multiple locations across the IDN to providers at different locations for the support of disease management. As discussed throughout this chapter, leading IDNs are pursuing a long-term strategy of developing an enterprise infrastructure for information integration. Such a strategy is necessary to accomplish true enterprise data integration, and required for any kind of advanced data analysis or decision support.

Some organizations, however, also pursue the use of Web browser–based technology to present clinicians with access to patient data from multiple legacy databases around the enterprise. This approach is attractive for several reasons:

- Use of a platform-independent application facilitates access to data from virtually any site with modem access (depending on security requirements).
- The browser application offers the opportunity to provide access in the absence of a well-developed, integrated information infrastructure.
- It is possible to channel feeds from multiple disparate systems to a single Web server, so virtual data integration can be accomplished in the absence of several core integration elements, such as a clinical data repository.
- It eliminates the need for IS support of the user desktop, unless this is required for other applications.
- Most attractive of all, these applications can be developed and implemented inexpensively and relatively quickly—their major advantage over implementation of vendor-based solutions.

A variety of factors motivated the organizations that have opted to develop Web-based access systems. One common feature was the perceived need to deliver access to data inexpensively and in the very near term—far sooner than would be possible through a major system implementation or overhaul. In one organization with a one-thousand-physician, multispecialty clinic associated with its university medical center, each clinic maintained separate medical records, and no straightforward mechanism existed for communicating clinical information among providers in the clinics or in the hospital. The IS department elected to take advantage of the predominant use of one transcription service by many physicians to build an interface from this system to an NT server where the dictated notes could be displayed as narrative text. The effort made available to providers large amounts of important clinical data in a short period. Another organization utilized a browser-based front end to replace rapidly an old store-and-forward system, at some cost savings and with increased functionality. It may become the front end for future clinical systems.

Another characteristic of some organizations pursuing browser-based technology is the need for a flexible application that can be tailored to its unique information needs. The specialists at the university hospital clinic practice just described had been unable to select a vendor system that met their diverse needs; the ability to customize the new browser application was a major selling point. A cancer research hospital chose to employ a Web-browser application to provide access to oncology protocols and to permit remote entry of highly specialized patient evaluation forms by study nurses in the field; such flexibility is not available in vendor products.

The principle hazards associated with use of the browser approach to providing data access are related to the fact that these applications are typically developed in-house by IS staff or interested users and therefore have all of the potential pitfalls of homegrown software. Chief among these is development around software applications, especially databases, that are not sufficiently robust to scale to the enterprise level. One organization we studied is realizing that it soon must arrest its rollout so that it can port all data to a better database platform. Some organizations have courted start-up Web-development groups but have found these organizations' lack of experience in health care to be a serious liability, or they have had concerns regarding the companies' viability and dependability.

IS Support for Referral Management.   Referral management in most settings today is equated with referral authorization: obtaining approval for a referral, according to payer-established rules. As IDNs begin to assume the financial risk for medical management, payer rules fall out of the equation and the IDN must establish internal guidelines for approval of referrals according to medical appropriateness.

We identified one IDN-sponsored initiative that stresses management based on medical appropriateness. This organization is in an intensely competitive metropolitan area and increasingly accepts full-capitation contracts from the major payers in the region. It has a large management services organization (MSO), within which approximately 30 percent of providers are owned by the IDN and the remainder rely, although not exclusively, on the MSO to negotiate contracts.

The organization believes, based on its IS capabilities and preliminary cost data, that it can reap the benefits of efficient management of care delivery under risk bearing. Its approach is to assume risk for targeted processes (such as medication subcapitation), patient groups (such as those with specific chronic conditions), and eventually, general capitated patient populations. It sees referral management as integral to this process, allowing it to extend its capacity for disease management across the continuum of care.

The IDN has built an application that is integrated closely with its enterprise systems, allowing it to import data—clinical, demographic, and insurance—that currently are captured elsewhere, thereby minimizing the amount of data entry required of clinicians. In addition, to guide the referral process it is building in referral-management rules based on both provider authorization rules (when appropriate) and medical appropriateness. These rules are determined by the MSO medical management department. The application permits on-line approval of many uncomplicated referrals, saving considerable clinician and patient time. The application is in the early pilot phase with a small number of owned physicians. Rollout will proceed to these physicians first, because they have enterprise workstations already installed, and then to nonowned affiliates. The latter may choose a variety of formats for receiving referral information, depending on the technical infrastructure.

The greatest difficulty encountered by the organization during the design phase was in obtaining consistent referral rules from the medical administration—specifically, learning from the administration precisely how it wanted the rules to operate. The task will become more complex as the application is rolled out more broadly, and IS will have to accommodate additional regional medical organizations, ten of which are represented within the MSO. It is likely that each of these will have different medical management rules and contract differences.

That the IDN was able to launch such an ambitious initiative is largely a result of the preexistence of integrated hospital-based information systems and the availability of unique resources in its strong in-house development group, who are experienced in the implementation of rules-based systems. The organization was also aided by the relatively tight integration of its providers under an MSO with significant contracting power. The MSO has substantial leverage with its providers, as well as payers, giving it a great advantage over many IDNs. In provider organizations that are not in an advanced stage of physician integration, referral management is far more challenging and likely will remain limited to authorization management for the immediate future.

The Importance of Clinical Informaticists

> *Best practices:* (1) Clinical informaticists should be leveraged by IS departments for their ability to act as highly effective clinician liaisons and their ability to promote standardization of clinical practice, with accompanying cost savings and quality improvement. (2) At those few institutions with a tradition of in-house development of clinical systems, the informaticist's main responsibilities could include system design and development, analysis of the effects of implementing these systems, publication of their findings, and leading efforts to standardize clinical practice.

As the vital importance and potential of advanced clinical information systems has become clear in recent years, so too has the necessity of formally incorporating experienced clinicians—particularly physicians—into IS leadership. All of the IDNs we studied made use of clinical informaticists in physician–end-user liaison roles; eight of the ten employed physicians part-time or full-time in IS.

Two of the study IDNs based at academic medical centers employed large informatics research groups. Physicians from these groups worked with IS to develop clinical systems in accordance with clinician needs and conducted research into the subsequent performance of these systems.

At most IDNs, however, the most common role for the clinical informaticist is that of liaison between IS and users. Although these individuals have played an important role from the first appearance of clinical systems, a recent trend has rendered their contribution vital. Organizations increasingly realize that some of the greatest value from the use of clinical information systems is obtained when the system is regularly used by physicians as a standard part of their workflow. Physician use of clinical systems increases the potential value of point-of-care decision support by an order of magnitude, because it allows the system to affect decisions before they are implemented and avoid unnecessary costs and potential harm. In the hospital, physician order entry presents the optimal opportunity in this regard. In the outpatient setting, advanced ambulatory medical records provide decision support to the physician user for each patient visit, and order entry can be incorporated into the ambulatory setting as well.

Generating physician interest in, and eventually obtaining their buy-in to, the implementation of such systems is essential to the success of these systems, because they directly alter the way physicians practice medicine. There is no substitute for a physician champion within IS to facilitate this process.

The CIO of one academic medical center–oriented IDN described the role of informaticists at that organization as critical to the maintenance of its ability to compete on the basis of clinical excellence as opposed to that of lower costs. "We must achieve A's in infrastructure and clinical systems in order to succeed," he said. The informaticists are essential to promoting the effective use of the organization's advanced clinical systems.

One of the IDNs employs a physician full-time with the title of medical director of information systems. He functions as a physician advocate and also oversees physician advisory committees for information systems. He has provided crucial liaison support as the organization pursues the large-scale rollout of an ambulatory medical record system to its owned physician practices.

Interestingly, the CIO forum discussion revealed differences of opinion among CIOs regarding the need for physician informaticists to continue to practice medicine. On the one hand, most participants felt that part-time clinical practice is essential for an informaticist's credibility with clinicians; those who do not practice are likely to be perceived as computer nerds rather than as "real doctors." On the other hand, one CIO has had success employing nonpracticing physicians and even nonphysician medical informaticists as site representatives for IS, performing an educational function and promoting clinical informatics and quality improvement efforts. His IDN formed a clinical integration group and hierarchy, with a clinical board for each service line, that serve to link clinical informaticists.

Participants predicted that organizations that are unable to field sufficient physician informatics leadership will be unable to implement and champion advanced systems and eventually will be consumed by competitors. Having more physician leaders also provides leverage for clinical IS development within an organization. Doubtless, the need for clinical informaticists varies according to the nature and size of each institution. Similarly, the extent to which a clinician-informaticist's credibility requires ongoing practice of medicine depends entirely on the culture and politics in each organization.

System Management

We analyzed four critical elements of IS management at the organizations in the study: standards, development partnerships, security, and advanced technology management.

Controlling IS Standards

Best practices: The method by which central control over enterprise standards is achieved should vary according to the structure and culture of the organization. Two techniques of controlling standards outside of the budgetary realm of IS are (1) purchasing department surveillance of all information technology–related purchase orders for standards conformance, according to uniform IS criteria; and (2) a graded approach to standards enforcement, with IS support and connectivity dependent on adherence to standards.

Controlling technical standards across the IDN is one of the most important functions performed by the enterprise IS department. Without adequate control of IS standards, enterprise communications—and associated efforts to operate the IDN as a coherent business entity—are seriously impaired, and resources must be diverted from strategic initiatives to support efforts to overcome barriers to linking nonstandard systems. IS departments should name an individual or group to be responsible for overseeing standards policies and for educating the organization about standards.

A common approach to controlling standards across the enterprise is to establish purchasing department policies requiring review of communications computer–related purchase orders for adherence to IS department standards. This approach has the advantage of providing surveillance over information technology purchases that do not appear in the IS department's standard budgeting process.

A more flexible approach to standards enforcement may be required in large organizations in which the IS department has limited control over some of the more loosely affiliated entities. In these cases, it may make sense to pursue a policy of dialogue and surveillance of the various environments so as to remain apprised of local IS initiatives and to be able to gauge users' needs for interoperability with other elements of the enterprise. One IDN takes such an approach, illustrated in Figure 9.5, requiring different levels of adherence to enterprise standards according to users' desire to obtain access to enterprise connectivity and data; departmental support is provided according to the extent to which systems adhere to enterprise standards. Another approach that appears to be gaining popularity in particularly challenging environments is to entice users to want to standardize because of the excellent support that is provided to all users of products that are compliant with the organization's standards.

Vendor Partnerships

> *Best practices:* The keys to successful vendor partnership include strong executive management support for the effort, adequate in-house technical expertise, and adequate in-house project management resources.

Vendor partnerships—in which software vendors and the organization's IS departments combine resources to address specific systems needs of the IDN—

FIGURE 9.5. LOCAL FREEDOM VERSUS CENTRAL CONTROL OF STANDARDS.

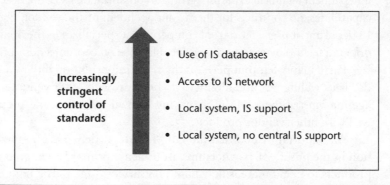

Increasingly stringent control of standards

- Use of IS databases
- Access to IS network
- Local system, IS support
- Local system, no central IS support

are an inescapable aspect of IDN information management today. Even organizations with large in-house informatics groups staffed by people who are experienced in clinical systems development are partnering with vendors to develop and implement enterprise systems such as enterprisewide patient identification or clinical data repositories.

The elements required for a successful vendor partnership include strong executive support for IS initiatives, project management resources, and in-house technical expertise. Solid executive backing is essential to enable the IS group to bargain aggressively and to terminate discussions or a pilot project—sometimes in the face of strong user support. Strong project management resources are necessary to ensure adherence to time lines and budgetary limitations; vendors should not be relied on to perform this function. In-house technical expertise is necessary to allow the IS department to reality-check vendor resources and recommendations. It may also prove invaluable if the vendor abandons support for the product, as happens occasionally.

One CIO characterized the traditional IDN-vendor relationship as one of "mutual assured destruction"—borrowing a phrase from Cold War nuclear strategy. In such a relationship, commitment is based on interdependence for survival, with the corollary that each partner is capable of severely damaging the other. The participant emphasized that relationships are evolving away from this tradition in some respects, but a careful examination of each party's motives and the subsequent alignment of incentives remains essential, and the vendor and IDN need not be permanently "married."

Indeed, maintaining a healthy degree of independence is good strategy. One organization from our study learned this when faced with abandonment of a strategic database project by the vendor. Ample technical resources allowed the IDN to take over the maintenance of the system. The tenuous financial footing of many current IS vendors makes this a particularly important consideration. One organization in our study had implemented an interesting approach to provide vendor-independent technical expertise. When his organization lacks the necessary in-house capabilities, he contracts for them—independent of the vendor. For example, the IS department uses an external company that specializes in the analysis of object-oriented technologies to perform due diligence on certain vendor products.

Participants felt that perhaps the most important quality in a potential vendor is its willingness and ability to do business with other vendors. The vendor's agenda must go beyond simply having its own product work—it must integrate well with other vendor products.

An important trend that the CIO forum participants observed is the transition in the nature of partnerships, from being primarily centered on delivery of products to being increasingly based on service. One participant suggested that consultants could take a more active role in educating vendors about the way they present their products and services to buyers. An example given was the lack of sensitivity to operational realities demonstrated by offering 8 A.M. to 5 P.M. support services in the "basic price" for mission-critical applications.

Management of Security and Confidentiality

Best practices: The use of the available technical security measures (for example, selective auditing of look-ups or frequent password changes), plus establishment, publication, and rigorous enforcement of confidentiality policies, can produce a culture of respect for issues of confidentiality.

We observed considerable variation among organizations' approaches to system security and protection of patient confidentiality. A number of organizations were notably remiss in developing and implementing a solid security policy. At these sites we encountered use of group IDs, passwords pasted on terminals, and lack of terminal time-outs that would permit virtually anyone access to confidential patient data. Staff at these sites were not satisfied with their existing security approaches; however, they certainly are close to the state of the practice in health care today. A recent study conducted by the National Research Council found similar practices in sites that had been specifically selected because they represented best practices.[7]

Several other organizations pursued rigorous implementation of technical security measures: regular review of audit trails on data access, frequent user-password changes, and terminal time-outs. One organization was implementing a more sophisticated approach to security management: a graded, user role–specific technology based on the nature of a user's participation in a patient's care. The system allows emergency overrides to permit access to data to other than the usual providers, but such overrides trigger an audit alert informing the IS department of the incident. Most important, however, the organizations that have chosen to implement technical security measures aggressively have followed up by publicizing these measures and by strictly enforcing their policies—including terminating the employment of individuals who have been found inappropriately accessing patient data. The clear publication and enforcement of such policies can help to create a culture of respect for security and confidentiality. It is fortunate that the industry is beginning to develop tools for assessing security levels and implementing improved practices.[7] (See guidelines published by the Computer-Based Patient Record Institute, available at http://www.cpri.org.)

Linkage of Technology and Business Goals

Control of Advanced Technology Initiatives

Best practices: (1) Organizations should have established policies for evaluation of new technologies, and these policies should be spelled out in the IS strategic plan; and (2) advanced technology evaluation should be the responsibility of a specific individual or group, who must ensure adherence to these policies.

A technology that is new to an organization presents both opportunity and risk. Although a new technology might, for example, extend the functionality of existing systems to new settings—as in the case of wireless devices in the hospital or clinic setting or the use of telemedicine to provide consultation over distances—it remains an unknown quantity until it is tested in the new environment. Problems subsequently encountered include unanticipated costs, lack of local technical expertise to support the system, and unpredictable capacity to interface with existing technologies.

For these reasons, IDNs should incorporate a strategy for managing advanced technology investments into their IS strategic plan. One study organization has appointed a technology review officer; two others have designated technology review committees that evaluate risks and benefits of candidate new technologies. One of these organizations has recently and successfully implemented a groupware system across the IDN and wireless workstations on inpatient wards.

New Technology Implementation: Business Case and Workflow Considerations

Best practices: When considering implementation of advanced technologies, careful attention should be paid to ensuring that (1) the implementation fits with the business environment and supports the organization's business goals, and (2) the new technology will integrate into the workflow at the target setting. Use of experienced clinician liaisons can be invaluable in facilitating this integration.

We observed two principle success factors for the successful implementation of new technologies in the workplace. First, the technology must address a business need of the IDN. Second, the implementation must be carried out with scrupulous attention to the workflow realities of the environment.

Telemedicine is an example of a technology—or more properly, a family of technologies for distance communications—whose theoretical advantages and practical limitations stand in stark contrast. In principle, telemedicine can facilitate distance consultation, providing physicians in remote settings with expert advice based on the availability to a consultant of transmitted images, both fixed and real-time, and of sound and electrical recordings and other forms of data.

Against this potential stands a series of significant limitations. First, regulations regarding reimbursement for telemedicine services are very much in flux. At the time of the study, reimbursement was available for only certain teleradiology consultations, and Medicare reimbursement for consultations was uncommon. The practice of distance medicine raises legal issues regarding practicing across state lines; theoretically, a physician who provides a consultation must be licensed in the state where the patient is evaluated. Most telemedicine programs have had their origins in government grant-funded projects, and most have not become self-supporting for the reasons mentioned earlier. Thus there have been few business success stories in telemedicine, although recent legislative initiatives may change this.

One of the participating IDNs developed a business plan for a telemedicine initiative that took these realities into consideration. The IS director reasoned that the organization's increasingly capitated environment presented an opportunity to profit from a form of care that is not traditionally reimbursed, if it offered cost savings compared with traditional care. Therefore, if telemedicine services for outpatients could obviate the need for hospitalization, a business case could be made for their use. The organization designed and piloted two programs aimed at assisting in the home care of recently discharged patients at high risk for readmission. The programs were designed to study the costs and outcomes of the alternative approach to care. The same organization ran a financially successful international telemedicine referral program (which of course was not subject to restrictions on reimbursement). The example illustrates the importance of proper attention to the business case for any new-technology initiative.

This example may be contrasted with another study participant, whose teleradiology system originated with federal grant money and whose planning was described by one senior executive as haphazard at best. At the time of our site visit, the system was not widely used for actual practice of medicine; several pilot projects were under development, and the value of this investment in support of specific business objectives was not clear.

Fit with workflow is an important consideration for any system implementation. A careful examination of existing workflow patterns is an essential part of planning for any installation and includes an assessment of the potential need to redesign elements of workflow in preparation for system implementation. These considerations are particularly important when considering implementation of a new technology that directly affects the end user—the chief objective of the new technology is precisely to change the way the user works.

We observed several examples of the implementation of wireless mobile workstations on inpatient wards among our study IDNs. The most successful implementation dealt directly with the challenge of changing end-user behavior. This organization implemented wireless workstations on the inpatient wards in its central hospital. The objective of the project was to increase physician use of the computer system and in particular to encourage physician order entry. The wireless project was conceived specifically to fit with the physicians' work patterns: they were in the habit of writing orders while walking from patient room to room. To facilitate the training process, an IS physician liaison (a registered nurse) accompanied physicians during rounds to acquaint them with the use and benefits of the system. This attention to fit with workflow successfully addressed a specific business goal, resulting in increased use of the hospital systems by physicians.

Conclusions

The observations gleaned from our study and presented in this chapter should be interpreted in the context of a rapidly evolving, highly heterogeneous industry, where true integration is the exception rather than the rule. The central themes can be summarized in ten "rules" for infrastructure management in integrated delivery systems, illustrated in Figure 9.1 and summarized as follows:

- The commitment of an organization's executive management to information systems as a strategic asset is an essential success factor for proper function of an IS department. Such commitment must be aggressively and continuously fostered by the CIO through educational and awareness-raising efforts.
- CIOs must be involved from the outset in planning for organizational change to allow them to position IS to facilitate enterprise integration processes.
- Predictions of the value of strategic initiatives should be based both on likely contributions to organizational strategic goals and on evidence of value demonstrated in other organizations. The task of "selling" the value of IS to executive management requires an intimate appreciation of the specific roles and views of individual executives and stakeholders.
- The organizations studied tend to concentrate effective governance among small groups of senior management. New organizational structures may help to confront the difficulties of cross-continuum care delivery and thereby address one of the most challenging aspects of IDN function, but there are no simple solutions to the inherent trade-off between accountability and flexibility in these matrix-managed organizations.
- IS support for processes of physician integration, particularly disease and referral management, will be essential to the long-term success of IDNs in the managed care environment.

- Clinical informaticists should be leveraged by IS departments for their ability to act as highly effective clinician liaisons and for their ability to promote standardization of clinical practice, with accompanying cost savings and quality improvement. Informaticists' primary responsibilities can include system design and development, rigorous analysis of the effects of implementing and using these systems and publication of their findings, and leading their peers in efforts to standardize clinical practice.
- The method by which central control over enterprise standards is achieved will vary according to the structure and culture of the organization, and the feasibility of centralized control may also vary depending on the stage of integration of the IDN.
- Keys to a successful vendor partnership include strong executive management support for the effort, adequate in-house technical expertise, and in-house project management resources. CIOs are increasingly concerned not simply with an application's track record but also with the vendor's capacity and willingness to work well with other vendors.
- The use of available technical security measures must be coupled with the establishment, publication, and rigorous enforcement of confidentiality policies to produce a culture of respect for confidentiality.
- Successful implementation of advanced technologies requires a clear linkage between the technology initiative and organizational business goals and careful attention to integration with workflow. Use of a clinician liaison can assist with this integration.

Notes

1. Nilson, J. T. "Fifteen Integration Challenges: What You Can Do to Smooth the Transition." *Healthcare Executive*, 1998, *13*, 21–24.
2. College of Healthcare Information Management Executives. *The H.I.S. Desk Reference: A CIO Survey.* Baltimore, Md.: HCIA, 1997.
3. Snodgrass, B. N. "Analyzing Business Processes with FEA." *ADVANCE for Health Care Executives*, 1997, *6*, 33–36.
4. Violino, B. "Return on Investment." *Information Week*, June 30, 1997, pp. 36–44.
5. Koch, C. "A Tough Sell." *CIO*, 1997, *10*, 74–86.
6. Computer-Based Patient Record Institute Work Group on CPR Systems Evaluation. *Valuing CPR Systems: A Business Planning Methodology.* Schaumburg, Ill.: Computer-Based Patient Record Institute, 1997.
7. Committee on Maintaining Privacy and Security in Health Care Applications of the National Information Infrastructure. *For the Record: Protecting Electronic Health Information.* Washington, D.C.: National Academy Press, 1997.

APPENDIX A: ATTRIBUTES OF AN INTEGRATED DELIVERY NETWORK

All organizations that consider themselves to be an "Integrated Delivery Network" are evolving toward increased integration of structure, clinical processes, basic operations, and information infrastructure. The following is an attempt to list the attributes of a highly integrated IDN. Please rate your IDN's integration status for each attribute on a range from 0 to 3, where:

0 = None (all local)
1 = Just beginning to integrate across settings
2 = We are somewhat there
3 = Totally integrated
? = I don't know

Check one answer for each bulleted item listed below:

Integrated Attributes	*Your IDN Rating*				
Structural	0	1	2	3	?
The health care services provided within the network include, at a minimum, primary care, specialty physician care, and inpatient care.	○	○	○	○	○
The IDN has one corporate mission statement and one business strategy.	○	○	○	○	○
A single chief executive and one board are accountable for all the component entities as a whole.	○	○	○	○	○
The IDN executive team includes senior executives who are accountable for the operational, financial, and clinical performance of the entire enterprise.	○	○	○	○	○
The IDN engages in single signatory contracting.	○	○	○	○	○
Each entity within the IDN can be placed on an organizational chart as belonging to the same unified organizational structure.	○	○	○	○	○
Management jobs are defined in terms of the IDN business objectives, which are reflected in performance measures and incentives.	○	○	○	○	○
JCAHO considers the organization a candidate for accreditation as a health care delivery network.*	○	○	○	○	○
Corporate products are defined along clinical/service/product lines that cross traditional settings.	○	○	○	○	○
There is identifiable leadership/responsibility for managing and improving cross-enterprise processes.	○	○	○	○	○
Financial incentives for component entities and participants (including physicians) are aligned.	○	○	○	○	○
The entity operates its own health plan (full risk for cost as well as quality).	○	○	○	○	○

* " … *a network is an entity that provides, or provides for integrated health care services to a defined population of individuals. ["A defined population"] is not necessarily a population enrolled in a health plan, it is simply the patient groups or community (ies) served by the system. A network offers comprehensive or specialty services and is characterized by a central structure that coordinates and integrates services provided by component organizations and practitioners participating in the network."*

Integrated Attributes	Your IDN Rating

	0	1	2	3	?

Operational Integration

Redundant corporate services and functions have been consolidated into a common process to gain effiencies and provide a common, integrated view of the performance of the business.	◯	◯	◯	◯	◯
Budgeting and financial statements are consolidated around corporate product lines rather than individual settings of care.	◯	◯	◯	◯	◯
A common process supports contracting with outside payers to provide cross-continuum services.	◯	◯	◯	◯	◯
Common credentialling, peer review, and medical staff development processes are in place across the IDN's component institutions.	◯	◯	◯	◯	◯
Service performance standards and policies and procedures that govern operations are centrally determined and universally applicable across the IDN.	◯	◯	◯	◯	◯
Human resources needs determination, recruitment, hiring, compensation, training, and scheduling are integrated into a common process that facilitates assignment of staff across settings.	◯	◯	◯	◯	◯

Clinical Integration

Practice standards enable providing one standard of care, regardless of where a member is treated.	◯	◯	◯	◯	◯
Members have to access to care via "one-stop shopping."	◯	◯	◯	◯	◯
Member care is coordinated seamlessly across care settings (including external contracted sites).	◯	◯	◯	◯	◯
Episodes of care can be tracked, and outcomes of care determined across settings.	◯	◯	◯	◯	◯
At any time, one team or person (primary care manager or case manager) has overall responsibility for coordinating each member's care and the member knows who the responsible party is and how to access care.	◯	◯	◯	◯	◯
Maintaining wellness of the population is an active part of the delivery system.	◯	◯	◯	◯	◯

Integration Attributes	Your IDN Rating

Information Integration

	0	1	2	3	?
There is single accountability for information management throughout the IDN.	○	○	○	○	○
Individual members and providers can be uniquely identified throughout the care settings of the IDN.	○	○	○	○	○
Care providers have access to any member information they need, regardless of where in the IDN a member appears seeking care.	○	○	○	○	○
Member registration is a coordinated process for the enterprise, whereby each member registers once and can notify the IDN once of changes in demographic information and be assured that the update is available anywhere in the organization that it is needed.	○	○	○	○	○
Members and payers can provide initial information and updates to information concerning insurance eligibility and coverage once and be assured that current information is available anywhere in the organization it is needed.	○	○	○	○	○
A single, unified problem list is maintained for each IDN member, reflecting input from direct care providers throughout the organization.	○	○	○	○	○
Multiple member services provided by different departments and/or settings can be scheduled in a coordinated way.	○	○	○	○	○
Staff at member access points throughout the IDN have information about each member's primary care location and manager, and can direct the member there, as appropriate.	○	○	○	○	○
Information to meet payer requirements for review is produced as a byproduct of care delivery and documentation.	○	○	○	○	○
Information tools are available to care providers at the point of service to guide decisions about "best practice" from the clinical and financial perspectives.	○	○	○	○	○
Primary care case managers and specialist providers are assisted in meeting payer requirements for authorizations and rules concerning duration and locations of care by having this information available at the point of service.	○	○	○	○	○
Physicians and other care providers in the IDN are able to communicate seamlessly with their colleagues regardless of the proximity of their offices or care settings.	○	○	○	○	○
Clinical practice managers are able to analyze costs and outcomes of care episodes that span multiple care settings within the IDN.	○	○	○	○	○
Risk managers are able to analyze utilization of services throughout the IDN by discrete member populations.	○	○	○	○	○
The IDN is able to produce common member statements and payer bills that combine services from all settings.	○	○	○	○	○

APPENDIX B: CHARACTERISTICS OF BENCHMARK SITES

Denominators for Comparing Organizations According to Size

We attempted to gather metrics that are more applicable to IDNs than the traditional denominators used for comparisons (such as number of inpatient beds). We hypothesized that revenues are a better gauge of IDN size than bed count. Revenues are representative of business across all settings; they represent business independent of hospital bed occupancy rate, and they are a common denominator for comparison with other industries. Although the small number of participating organizations precludes reaching statistically significant conclusions, the data gathered appear to support the hypothesis that operating revenues is a useful denominator for comparing IDNs. The following figures utilize revenues, number of users, and number of workstations as denominators to characterize the participants.

- The organizations studied ranged from $350 million to $2.6 billion in total revenues, as depicted in Figure B.1.
- The number of networked workstations in the study organizations ranged from 1,000 to 23,000, as illustrated in Figure B.2.
- The number of users ranged from 3,500 to 20,000 at the participating IDNs, as shown in Figure B.3.

FIGURE B.1. REVENUES OF IDNS PARTICIPATING IN STUDY.

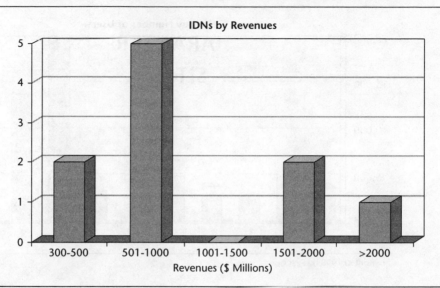

IDNs by Revenues

Revenues ($ Millions)

FIGURE B.2. WORKSTATIONS IN PLACE AT IDNS PARTICIPATING IN STUDY

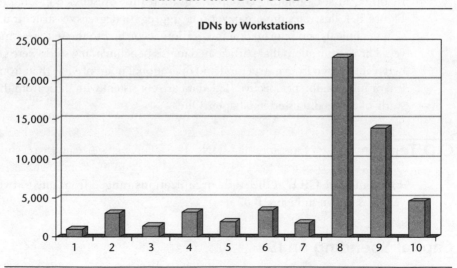

IDNs by Workstations

FIGURE B.3. REVENUES OF IDNS PARTICIPATING IN STUDY.

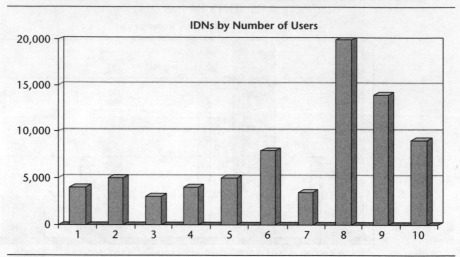

IDN Degree of Integration

We studied the stage of integration of the ten organizations using the Scottsdale Institute/First Consulting Group Integration Index discussed in Chapter One. Figure B.4 illustrates the organizations' aggregate degrees of structural, operational, clinical, and information integration according to the self-assessment survey. The organizations that participated in this benchmarking study were generally better integrated from a structural and operational point of view than from a clinical or information perspective. The data are consistent with those from the larger study of IDNs discussed in Chapter One.

CIO Tenure

The tenure of CIOs at the study organizations ranged from one to twenty-six years, as shown in Figure B.5.

Capital Spending on IS

Examination of our study participants' capital expenditures on information systems yielded several interesting observations. On average, our participants devoted

FIGURE B.4. SELF-ASSESSED STUDY OF INTEGRATION REPORTED BY IDNS PARTICIPATING IN STUDY.

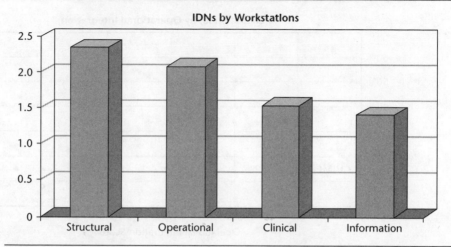

IDNs by Workstations

FIGURE B.5. AVERAGE TENURE OF CIOS.

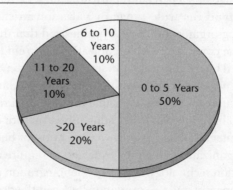

FIGURE B.6. CAPITAL INVESTMENT IN IS (PERCENTAGE) BY OPERATIONAL INTEGRATION.

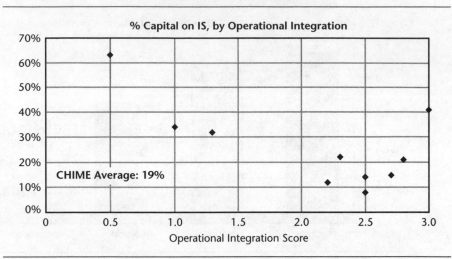

26 percent of their capital spending to information systems. This exceeds the industry average of 19 percent reported in the 1997 CHIME CIO survey. To better understand the wide range of variation in capital spending among the participating organizations, we hypothesized that these figures should be interpreted in the context of each organization's current level of operational integration, assessed by the Integration Index (such as existence of consolidated corporate functions, support for cross-continuum processes, and consolidated human resource functions). Organizations that are well integrated operationally might be expected to have more of an existing infrastructure in place, or else have established nonintegration technology workarounds for business processes; less well integrated organizations might be expected to require a greater capital investment in information technology as part of the integration process.

The apparent inverse correlation between the degree of operational integration and capital investment in information systems shown in Figure B.6 supports our hypothesis. As the graph illustrates, the organizations that invested less than 20 percent of their capital budget on information systems were among the most highly operationally integrated. Conversely, the organization with the largest percentage capital expenditure for information systems was the least operationally integrated. Thus the data suggest that the appropriateness of capital investment in information systems should be considered in the context of each organization's degree of operational integration.

Operating Budget Expenditures for IS

Figure B.7 shows the operating budgets of the participating organizations' information as a percentage of the total IDN operating budget. Interestingly, our participants had a lower average percentage of operating budget expenditure than the 1997 CHIME mean (2.6 percent versus 3.6 percent).

FIGURE B.7. IS OPERATING BUDGET AS A PERCENTAGE OF TOTAL OPERATING BUDGET, BY REVENUES.

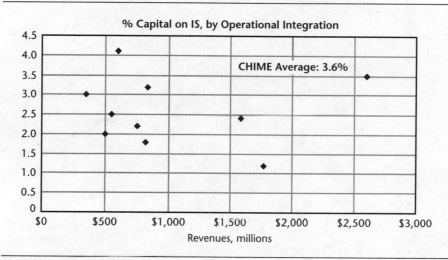

INDEX